I0796706

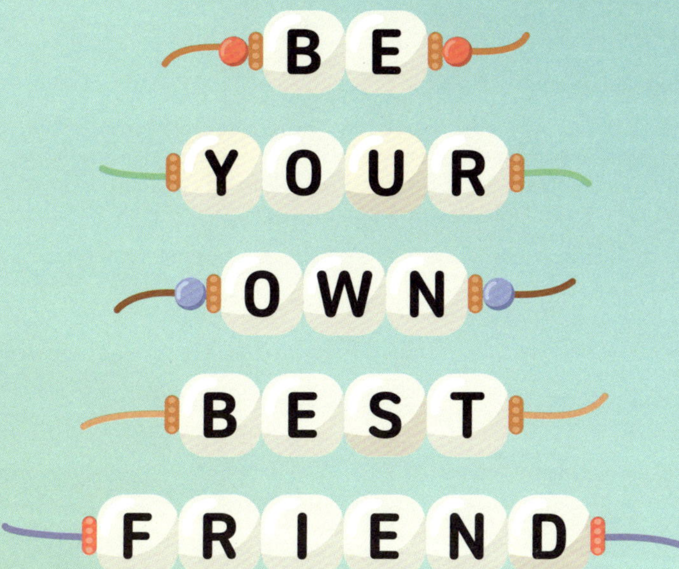
BE
YOUR
OWN
BEST
FRIEND

First published 2025

Exisle Publishing Pty Ltd
C/o Shortland Chartered Accountants Ltd, Level 9, 51 Shortland Street, Auckland 1010, New Zealand
PO Box 864, Chatswood, NSW 2057, Australia
www.exislepublishing.com

Copyright © 2025 in text: Nicola Lincoln

Nicola Lincoln asserts the moral right to be identified as the author of this work.

All rights reserved. Except for short extracts for the purpose of review, no part of this book may be reproduced, stored in a retrieval system or transmitted in any form or by any means, whether electronic, mechanical, photocopying, recording or otherwise, without prior written permission from the publisher.

A CiP record for this book is available from the National Library of New Zealand.

ISBN 978-1-923011-29-8

Designed by Bee Creative
Photography courtesy of Unsplash
Typeset in PT Serif, 11pt
Printed in China

This book uses paper sourced under ISO 14001 guidelines from well-managed forests and other controlled sources

10 9 8 7 6 5 4 3 2 1

Disclaimer

This book is a general guide only and should never be a substitute for the skill, knowledge and experience of a qualified medical professional dealing with the facts, circumstances and symptoms of a particular case. The nutritional, medical and health information presented in this book is based on the research, training and professional experience of the author, and is true and complete to the best of their knowledge. However, this book is intended only as an informative guide; it is not intended to replace or countermand the advice given by the reader's personal physician. Because each person and situation is unique, the author and the publisher urge the reader to check with a qualified healthcare professional before using any procedure where there is a question as to its appropriateness. The author, publisher and their distributors are not responsible for any adverse effects or consequences resulting from the use of the information in this book. It is the responsibility of the reader to consult a physician or other qualified healthcare professional regarding their personal care. This book contains references to products that may not be available everywhere. The intent of the information provided is to be helpful; however, there is no guarantee of results associated with the information provided.

BE YOUR OWN BEST FRIEND

A Teen's Guide to Self-Empowerment

NICOLA LINCOLN

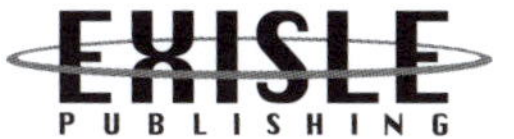

Praise for Nicola Lincoln:

'Nicola Lincoln has written an excellent guide for teens discussing the relevant issues and problems which teens struggle with. *Be Your Own Best Friend* includes resources and actionable suggestions that utilize mindfulness, empowerment, and positive affirmations to help teens practice proactive solutions to improve their mental health. Written in a way that speaks directly to teens, *Be Your Own Best Friend* is a book that I would share with any teen who needs guidance and supportive resources.'

KRISTIE THOMPSON, PH.D., LP, BCBA-D (LICENSED PSYCHOLOGIST AND BOARD CERTIFIED BEHAVIOUR ANALYST), NC, USA

'Nicola provides a comprehensive guide to help young people navigate their wellbeing from a holistic perspective. Her warmth and sincerity can be felt when reading this book and she provides engaging and easy to follow content on a wide variety of topics. *Be Your Own Best Friend* has many helpful "hands on" practical tools for teens, real-life examples and step-by-step guidance. It's great to have a book I can recommend to the teenagers I work with; I would highly recommend this to any young person going through the ups and downs of adolescence.'

DR MADELEINE HAEREWA (CHILD AND ADOLESCENT PSYCHOLOGIST), AUCKLAND NEW ZEALAND

"I have read this book and loved it! It is a great resource for young people. It encompasses a holistic approach to mental and emotional wellbeing. It provides young people with comprehensive information and a variety of practical tools to cope when facing challenges in life. By reading this book young people can gain skills that will help at any age. I certainly learned from reading it.

It is an easy read, and I think the author has captured her audience perfectly. I do love all the quotes. I will be buying a copy for my office to have to hand to support my work with young people."

ANDREA CURTIS, REGISTERED PSYCHOLOGIST, GUIDANCE COUNSELLOR AND DIRECTOR OF WELLBEING, AUCKLAND, NEW ZEALAND

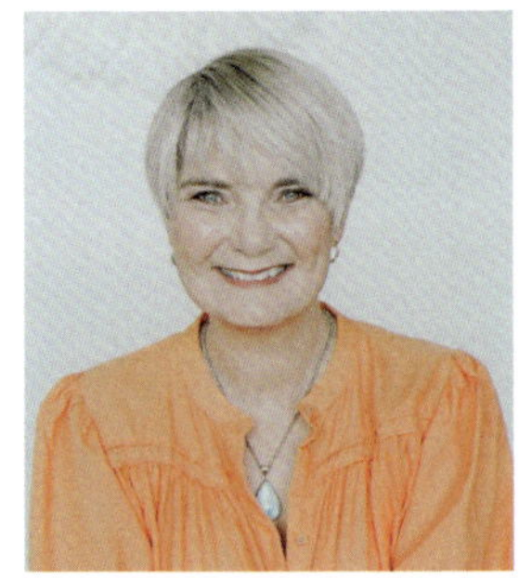

Nicola Lincoln is a Kiwi who travelled around the world when she was younger, returning to New Zealand to start a family and set up her wellness clinic.

She is a qualified naturopath and medical herbalist with sixteen years of clinical experience. Nicola received her Bachelor of Health Science (Complimentary Medicine) from the Charles Sturt University in Sydney, and she is also a Reiki Master Teacher, a Board Member of Reiki NZ Org., a PSYCH-K® Facilitator, spiritual mentor and author. She uses a holistic approach to healing on all levels of self — physically, mentally, emotionally and energetically. She has successfully helped many clients over the last sixteen years, having a passion for alternative therapies and mental health.

She has owned and run her own multidisciplinary wellness centre, practising naturopathy, Reiki and PSYCH-K® as well as teaching Reiki and various other workshops. She still sees clients of all ages for all health concerns, but her passion is helping young and old to manage their mental health. As well as running her clinic, she has supervised the naturopathic students at the South Pacific College of Natural Medicine in Auckland.

Nicola lives in Auckland, New Zealand, with her husband, two teenagers and her golden retriever.

'I felt drawn to write this book for a number of different reasons. Yes, it's my passion to help people live a healthy, fearless life, not being ruled by expectations and judgements, but mostly, it was due to my personal journey with my teen daughter. Her courage, wisdom and heartbreak dealing with this world through her lens of dyslexia, ADHD and anxiety, which ultimately steered her to self-harming, was my driving force to write something simple and user-friendly to help young people going through their own various emotional and mental health concerns.'

Praise for *Be Your Own Best Friend*:

'The stories of other teenagers fighting their own reminders is a gentle reminder that I am not so alone and also provides me with the reminder that we never know what other people are going through. Nicola's book acts as a kind reminder that we not only need to be kind to others, but also ourselves and to fight for peace and happiness every day, while showing ourselves grace in times of struggle. Nicola's book gave me hope.'

— AVA, 17

'Reading stories of real people and their experiences makes the things I deal with every day feel that much easier, knowing I'm not alone.'

— IZZY, 18

I would like to dedicate this book to:

My beautiful girl — you inspire me every day with your innate wisdom and courage.

And my gorgeous boy — thank you for being her rock. You are amazing.

I love you both to the stars and back again.

Contents

Note to Self

Be Kind to yourself

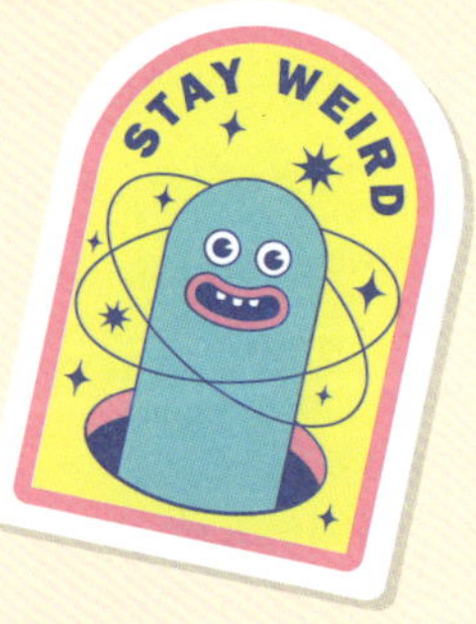

STAY CALM

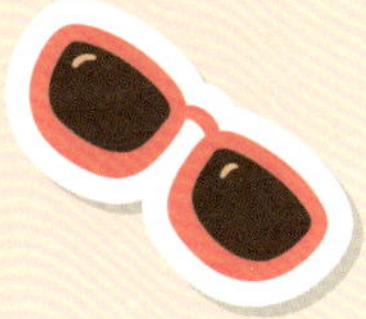

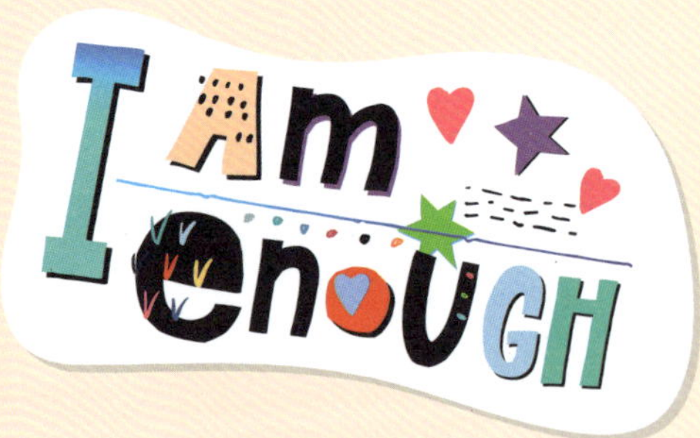

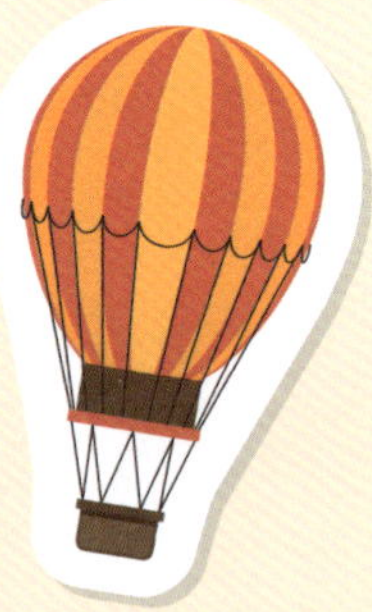

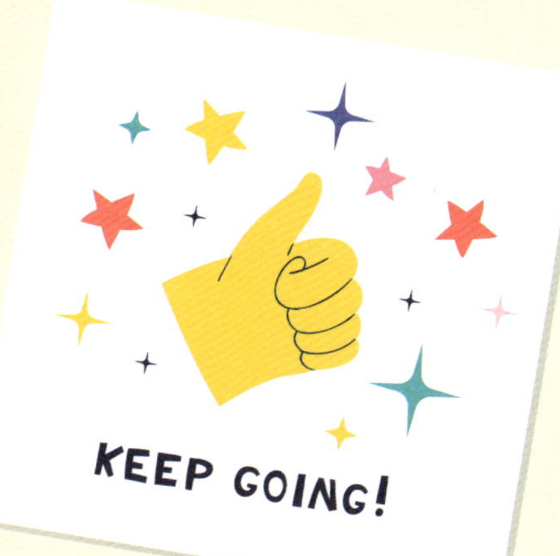

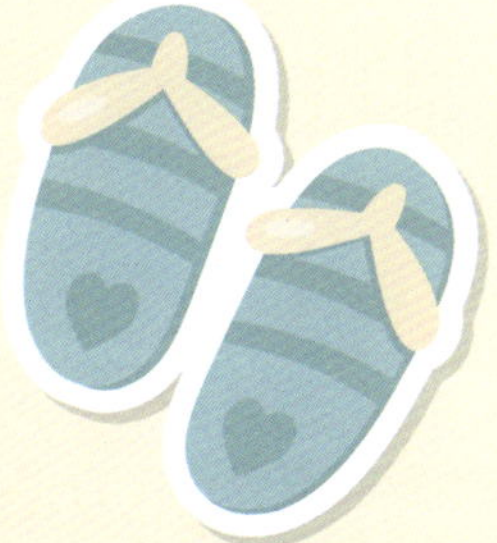

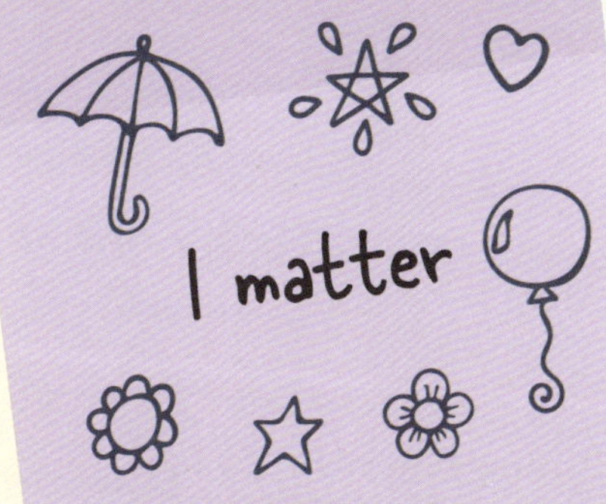

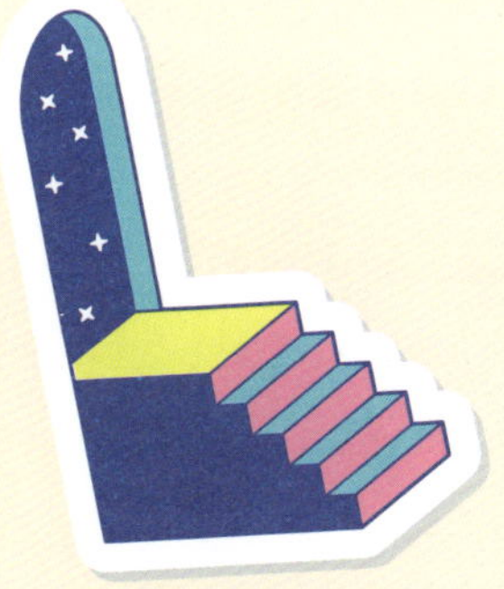

I AM
DESERVING

Note from Nic

If we were to meet and chat for the first time, I would most likely say to you:

> *'Who you are and what you know, in this moment, is enough. You are enough right now and you matter.'*

You are not defined by someone else's perception of you, but through your own beliefs, thoughts and feelings. And, if you are in pain, feeling angry, sad, hurt, worried, lost or lonely, the good news is, you have the ability to make choices and take action, to mend them. *Be Your Own Best Friend: A Teen's Guide to Self-Empowerment* provides the little daily steps to reimagine who and how you want to be. No one but you can do this. You are your own best counsel in all things relating to you. No one gets to judge or comment as they do not walk in your shoes each day.

Sure, others can certainly help, and it is important to feel like we belong and have trusted people in our lives. If feelings and thoughts become too overwhelming, it is a good idea to reach out to a family member, teacher, coach, school counsellor, psychologist or your GP. Ultimately, though, it is up to each of us to recognize when we need support and if we will act upon their advice — to be our own best friend.

With this book, you can read right through or dip in and out, picking and choosing what interests you to build your own personal, holistic, mental and emotional wellbeing toolkit. The aim is to have a range of tools to help you construct your day accordingly, as each day changes and evolves. Nothing stays the same — even the feelings you are experiencing now will evolve.

Each section is designed to empower you with a sense of control over your own thoughts, experiences, energy and lifestyle — when they are in alignment, this creates a healthy foundation for good mental wellbeing.

Scattered throughout the book are true stories from various teens describing their journeys through a variety of emotional and mental health concerns and behaviours. They were happy to share with you what they found helpful so far in their lives. Their names have been changed, so they remain confidential.

'Just when the caterpillar thought the world was ending, she became a butterfly.'

—BARBARA HAINES HOWETT

The INNER COACH Toolkit

1.

Self-Love

'How you love yourself is how you teach others to love you.'

—RUPI KAUR

Self-love is essential for good mental health. How we view ourselves is the very foundation all our thoughts, decisions and actions stem from, affecting every part of our lives.

It is not being conceited to put yourself first, to stand up for what you believe in if you do so with openness and kindness. It is important to value who you are, acknowledging your worth. There will always be someone who does not see it — but do not let it be you! If you want others to see your worth, you need to see it in yourself first.

Stop and think for a moment about how you talk to yourself. Are your words encouraging, compassionate and kind, or are they constantly chastising, judging and criticizing?

Believe it or not, it is you who has control over what the inner voice gets to say. You have the power to change the inner critic to that of an inner coach.

No one is born with an inner critic. Over time, the people in our lives express what they believe we can and cannot do, say or be according to their perceptions. Their words, expectations and judgements form our inner voice, which, in some cases, may be detrimental if they make us feel we are not good or worthy enough.

Changing our inner dialogue to empowering and caring thoughts starts the process of self-love, helping us to accept ourselves and other relationships, so they too can be filled with the same healthy, respectful boundaries.

For example, people pleasing is different from having a genuine connection or friendship because it requires us to betray parts of who we are, or to put our own needs and wants aside. This can eventually lead to feelings of being taken advantage of, resentment and anxiety as we try to suppress our own true feelings.

Do not underestimate the power of walking away — it can do you a lot of good! Walk away from those people who choose not to see your worth. Walk away from judgemental people who do not know the struggles you are facing or what you have been through. Walk away from those people you always have to please in order to be seen. Most importantly, choose to walk away from guilt, shame, self-doubt and fear — they do not determine who you are or your journey.

If you are in a friend group that has you doubting yourself or feeling like you're not quite good enough, then it's time to let them go. Whether they make you feel this way on purpose or not becomes irrelevant. Removing yourself from them lessens your inner doubtful dialogue as you're not around them anymore and, with that, your feelings start to recover. The easiest way to feel better is to surround yourself with better people, and become your own best friend.

Being private, not telling everyone everything about your life, is also okay as it is self-care. Sadly, a lot of people don't actually care and some may even secretly want you to fail. Your feelings of worth and belonging are not conditional upon or negotiated with other people. Those feelings need to be fostered and come from within.

If doubts become ongoing, they may lead to low self-esteem. Often those with low self-esteem find self-love difficult as they lack confidence in themselves and their abilities, becoming less resilient to others' criticisms.

No matter how badly you may view yourself or what your inner voice chirps, you have the ability to change your thought processes with a little understanding as to why you think a certain way in the first place. As with understanding, it gives you the power to change, adapt or release any limiting beliefs or intrusive thoughts, and replace them with empowering ones.

It is important to do this, as if we do not value, respect and love ourselves, it will affect every decision we make!

'A bird gets up every morning and sings its own song. It does not wait to hear what other birds are singing, nor does it look to see if another bird is getting more notice. It knows its song innately and sings. This is nature; knowing your song.'

—MICHELLE OKA DONER

The more we can sing our own song, that is, be ourselves and love doing so, not being influenced by other people's songs or others' expectations about how we should sing, the easier, simpler and more content our life may become.

Okay, so how can we get to that place where we can sing our own song and love it? The best step is to build a little self-assurance into our attitude and not be afraid to take some pride in ourselves.

We can do this by developing our self-esteem and resilience, understanding how our beliefs shape our thoughts, and using affirmations to change our inner critic to our inner coach. All these are talked about in the next sections.

2.

Self-Esteem

'Care about what other people think and you will always be their prisoner.'

—LAO TZU

Low self-esteem can develop in anyone who experiences challenging events that knock their confidence and feelings of self-worth. For instance, being bullied, having learning difficulties, unhappy childhood, relationship breakdowns, financial hardship or a traumatic event, to name just a few.

Those with low self-esteem often lack self-assurance in themselves and their abilities as they may feel inadequate, incompetent, unloved or are afraid of letting other people down. All these feelings impact and reinforce all mental health concerns.

If you are judging yourself harshly or think negatively about yourself regularly, you may have low self-esteem.

Here are some tips that can help:

- Ask a couple of trusted friends to write a paragraph about you and each other. Separately, you all write down why you like each person, including their qualities you admire. Reading their comments about you can help to see yourself from a different, more positive, perspective.
- Limit comparing yourself to others. *No one* is perfect or has the perfect life. Life's ups and downs affect everyone at various times in their lives — they just don't post about it on social media as it would ruin your perception of them. You do you!
- Practise self-acceptance, who you are in this moment. Everyone messes up or regrets something they said or did. Don't beat yourself up — rather be kind to yourself, acknowledging that you are always learning and evolving, and can do things differently if there is a next time.
- Develop positive relationships with family and friends. If you do not feel valued, respected or cared for by someone, it's time to talk with them about how you feel.
- Start accepting compliments. If you have low self-esteem this can be difficult, as a compliment often contradicts how you see yourself. Rather than going straight to a dismissive

reply, try simply saying 'thank you'. Let your brain hear that a few times, as it will start to make a new belief based on the praise.

- Do things that make you like yourself. Engage in activities you can be proud of, that make you feel good about yourself. Try a part-time job where you feel appreciated for your efforts, or do some voluntary or charity work. Helping others, doing something creative or completing a project are good ways to feel proud of yourself, of what you did, gave or achieved. Then make sure you acknowledge and praise yourself for doing so.
- The things you admire and value in others are the things already within yourself. Start recognizing and cultivating these positive aspects.
- To increase your confidence, use good posture. Standing up tall and spreading out your body makes it take up more space, providing the feeling and impression of confidence.
- Keep a journal of all the positive things you have achieved. Recent achievements to past ones, small and large. It's a great way to remind yourself you have been successful before, and know you can be again.

3.

Resilience

Resilience is the ability to bounce back from and positively adapt to the ongoing challenges in our lives. It is the level of ability we have to endure those difficult times.

People with high levels of resilience consider themselves to have high levels of wellbeing. Having high energy levels makes it easier to bounce back from adversity.

All symptoms of poor mental health are a signal that something is out of whack, trying to tell us something. If how we feel about a situation versus how we act towards it are not in alignment, this can lead to feelings of worry and stress, as our thoughts and actions are not united.

> **Be aware of your own beliefs and values. Ensure you live in accordance with them in all areas of your life — be true to yourself.**

Taking a stance against a situation that is not in accordance with our values will naturally build our resilience and confidence as we adapt to the adverse situation. This starts the process of taking back control of our environment, which positively affects our thoughts and feelings.

For instance, choosing to let go of a friendship that keeps you constantly on tenterhooks is a positive stance moving forward. Or if a friend decides they don't want to continue a relationship with you, rather than being too upset or hurt, try to stay positive and say to yourself, 'Okay, I know my worth, so one day, if they realize it too, they will come back wanting to be friends again, and I will get to choose if I want that.'

Be aware of your opinions and how they may be received by others. This allows you to cope better when people have differing opinions to your own. For example, when you stop judging and criticizing yourself harshly, it builds your self-esteem and self-worth. This makes it easier to let go of any negative feelings when others judge or criticize you harshly. They will start to flow over you rather than drowning you in feelings of inadequacy.

Build your own personal resilience toolkit. Make a list of your core values and beliefs. Add your strengths, skills and resources. Start the list with, 'I am ...', 'I can ...' and 'I have ...'. It's a good reminder of who you truly are. Take time to review it occasionally, as it will evolve as you do.

4.

Empowering Beliefs

'The world is nothing but my perception of it. I see only through myself. I hear only through the filter of my story.'

—BYRON KATIE

Our brain has two parts: the conscious and subconscious minds. We live 95 per cent of our life from our subconscious (below consciousness) and only 5 per cent from our conscious mind.

In the 5 per cent of conscious time, we are totally present; making intentional decisions, and we are at our most creative, that is, we are totally aware of what we are doing.

Incredibly, this means, for 95 per cent of our life, we are effectively on auto pilot! We are acting and thinking automatically based on our *past* history in the *present* moment.

Our subconscious is like a library that stores records on everything we have observed, experienced and learned. This forms the basis of all our beliefs, values and thoughts about life, which we will always automatically act from.

A large part of this was formed when we were a young child, learning the rules of life from our family, friends and teachers and how to fit in and feel valued.

Some beliefs are empowering and help us, like 'I like trying new things', while others are limiting or keep us stuck, like 'I'm not good enough'. We will always react and think based on those subconscious beliefs and records, whether rightly or wrongly.

If what we believe determines our thoughts and what we think generates our feelings, affecting our mood and decisions, then this makes *looking at our beliefs very important* to help us create the life we want.

Here are some tips to work out if you have any self-limiting beliefs, followed by possible ways to start viewing them differently:

- Look at where you are struggling in your life, such as relationships or at something you believe you cannot do like school work. Either way, there will be a belief that is *not* supporting what you are trying to achieve.
- Take a moment to identify exactly what it is you believe about yourself that is making you think a certain way, aggravating the areas you are struggling with. Think about why you believe it. Where does it come from? Then

consider, does the belief still feel appropriate and does the reason for it still sound credible to you?

- Write your story so far. Make a few notes about your life, a few paragraphs to a couple of pages on the ups and downs or struggles. You could even keep a journal to see if there are any patterns of behaviour that arise in various situations. For more on journalling see page 74.

  Read your notes or journal back several times. As you do, note what thoughts and feelings come to the surface and highlight any common themes. Take note of what circumstances surrounded these experiences. This provides clues about the limiting beliefs you may have formed.

- Imagine your friend was struggling with the same thing you are. What advice would you give them? Could you then take on board that same advice and encouragement? We are very good at seeing our friend's capabilities but rather poor at seeing our own.

- Think about a time when you did something with complete confidence. Look at why you felt that way, what you were doing and the situation. Then ask yourself, could you take that same confidence and use it now in your current situation?

When you understand what your self-limiting beliefs are, the next step is to change them into empowering ones, setting up new records your subconscious mind can work from. Basically, taking an unhelpful belief and converting it to a helpful one. A good way to do this is to use affirmations, as they are powerful statements to re-train and re-programme your brain.

'Keep your beliefs positive because:

Your beliefs become your thoughts.

Your thoughts become your words.

Your words become your actions.

Your actions become your habits.

Your habits become your values.

Your values become your destiny.'

—MAHATMA GANDHI

5.

Affirmations

'Change the way you see things, and the things you see will change.'

—DR WAYNE DYER

Your mind will believe what you constantly tell it, so please tell it you are smart, fearless and that you have what it takes!

Affirmations are a way to do this as they re-train and re-programme our subconscious through auto suggestion. An affirmation is a declaration, which when repeated over and over again, positively acts on our emotions and speaks directly to our subconscious mind to start thinking differently.

Affirmations are the repetitive words we say daily, like 'I am happy' over and over, until eventually we start to feel happier without having to say the words any more. As like attracts like, it is a powerful way to attract what we want into our lives. See tools on manifesting on page 78.

To work out what might be an appropriate affirmation, we first need to understand why we are feeling the way we do and what is triggering our mental health concerns. It could be due to a limiting belief (see Empowering Beliefs on page 10), a traumatic past event or an ongoing challenging situation.

Once we know the trigger or reason, our affirmation will be the *opposite* of it. For example, if someone made us feel we do not deserve love, the affirmation to counteract this belief is to repeatedly say to ourselves, 'I am worthy of love'. If we feel we are not good enough, it would be 'I am enough'.

Write your own affirmation

Here are the steps to write your own specific affirmation. There is a list of general affirmations you may like to try at the end of this section as well.

1. Start your statement with one of the following: 'I am ...', 'I have ...', 'I can ...', 'I believe ...' or 'I deserve ...'

   Starting a statement with 'I am ...' is powerful. Our subconscious interprets any statement starting with 'I am' as a command, a directive to make something happen.

2. Keep it in the first person and in the present tense. It's about you, not someone else. Describe what you want, as if you already have it right now. For example:

- Incorrect: ‘I am going to be happy’ or ‘I will be happy’.
- Correct: ‘I am happy.’

3. Use positive words to affirm what you want. For example:

   - Incorrect: ‘I am *no* longer afraid of change.’
   - Correct: ‘I embrace change in my life.’

4. The more meaningful it is, the better. Use one or two dynamic emotional words that describe what you would be *feeling* as if you had already achieved your desired outcome. Examples of words include joyfully, peacefully, calmly, lovingly, happily, successfully, proudly, effectively and enjoying.

   - For example: ‘I embrace change in my life with openness and curiosity.’

5. Keep it short, as your subconscious finds that easier to remember correctly.
6. Be specific — vague statements produce vague results.

How to use an affirmation

Once you have your affirmation, now it’s time to use it. It could feel silly doing so, but it is still worth doing; hence, there are a couple of options to try out. It is recommended to do one or more of the below for three weeks, but do it until you feel the desired outcome has been achieved.

1. Repeat it out loud three times in a row, several times throughout the day.

   Please persist, even if it feels awkward — as the more you do, the more your subconscious mind takes note and starts creating the new belief based on what it is hearing. This is how auto suggestion works.

2. A quick, powerful way for the belief to take hold is to say it while looking in a mirror. Look yourself in the eye and say the affirmation several times.

3. A comfortable way is to write the affirmation down 50 times on a piece of paper, saying it in your head as you write it. Do this daily.

4. A really easy way is to listen to affirmations or a meditation filled with positive words as you go to sleep. Put your headphones on, hit play and relax. You don't have to concentrate on what's being said, just relax and fall asleep as it continues. The soothing or inspiring information (depending on what you choose to listen to) will be recorded straight into your subconscious mind, creating new positive beliefs.

Affirmations to try

If you are not sure what would be good for you to say, here are some statements to get you started. Pick what feels right for you.

- 'I trust and believe in my ability to manage my life experiences.'
- 'I am deserving of love, happiness and joy.'
- 'I am worthy, wonderful and wise.'
- 'I am open to new experiences.'
- 'I believe in me and I am enough.'
- 'I am confident, happy and healthy.'
- 'I am competent, smart and able.'
- 'I am growing and changing for the better.'
- 'I dare to allow my visions and dreams to come true.'
- 'I expect the best and I always get what I expect.'
- 'I am unable to change another person – they are who they are, and I accept and love myself for who I am.'
- 'It is okay to be different from others; I am a unique person, as all are.'
- 'My body is unique and beautiful, and it doesn't need to look like anyone else's.'
- 'I am grateful for my [insert body part] as it can [insert what it can do for you].' For example, 'I am grateful for my nose as it can smell lovely things that make me feel happy.'
- 'I am more than any hurtful words thrown my way.'

- 'I choose to define myself, rather than through the words and beliefs of others.'
- 'I am deserving of fairness and kindness.'
- 'I embrace [insert the healing therapy] as a step towards my healing.' For example, 'I embrace counselling as a step towards my healing.'
- 'I forgive myself for believing I have to hold anger when I am bullied.'
- 'I forgive myself for believing it is my fault when I am bullied.'
- 'Me having more happiness is good for the world.'
- 'Me having more success is good for the world.'
- 'Me having more money is good for the world.'

6.

The Placebo Effect

Our mind, through its thoughts, constantly affects and directs our body, allowing us to become the chemist of our own blood. This is why the placebo effect is so powerful. It happens when someone has hope they will get better and believes what they are doing will make it so. In other words:

> **The body follows what the mind is thinking.**

This is what you see in clinical trials. For example, in a clinical trial for a new drug, say an anti-depressant medication, there are usually three controlled groups. One group gets the actual medication, one gets a placebo or 'sugar pill' that looks like a normal medical drug and the last group receives nothing, as they are the control group to be measured against.

When someone in a clinical trial receives the placebo pill, they are unaware of this, as it looks like any other type of medication. They think they are given the anti-depressants, and accept, believe and surrender, allowing the 'pill' to improve their mental wellbeing.

Their brain follows their emotional belief and their nervous system then creates the physical chemicals, like serotonin and endorphins, in their body that matches the belief. Healing occurs as depression recedes, even though they have only taken the sugar pill.

> **It is the power of their belief, attitude and expectation that they are being helped that allows their body to reflect that belief and healing starts.**

What is the consequence of negative thinking and beliefs on the body? Sadly, the feelings of dis-harmony result in 'dis-ease' physically, mentally or emotionally. Therefore, using tools like affirmations, building your resilience and self-esteem, setting up positive beliefs *all help to make the best chemistry in your body that lifts your mood and calms your nervous system and stress levels, which gives you better mental and emotional health.*

The HEALTHY BEHAVIOURS Toolkit

7.

Unhealthy Coping Habits

'Your hardest times often lead to the greatest moments in your life. Keep going.'

—JOKER INSPIRATION

When feelings of anxiety, doubt, depression, low self-esteem or intrusive, harmful thoughts are not managed, they can become overwhelming to the point where it is possible to feel numb, invisible or that everything is pointless or hopeless.

If these feelings are not resolved or are suppressed long enough, they can create an emotional void, the feeling of 'I don't care'. When we no longer care about anything, we can become disconnected from everything and everyone in our lives.

It is a way of protecting ourselves against these terrible feelings. The issue with this is that it stops both the bad from hurting us and the good from helping us.

This void is an invitation for action and it wants to be filled. Unfortunately, it is often done so with unhealthy coping behaviours, like alcohol and recreational drug use, detrimental eating behaviours or self-harming. They may temporarily make us feel better, giving a sense of having something within our control, but afterwards, they often lead to feelings of shame, regret or guilt, which reinforce all the original unpleasant emotions about ourselves and our life.

Using drugs and alcohol to numb difficult feelings and thoughts is not a permanent solution. Their effects on the body and mind are detrimental and the numbness doesn't last, allowing all the pain and angst to return. The desire to escape these feelings by using drugs or alcohol may lead to dependency and addiction. This comes at a cost — not just financially, but to your emotional and physical wellbeing too.

Drugs and alcohol both affect people in different ways. Some people are more sensitive to their effects and some experience the complete opposite to the expected high or euphoric sensation.

For safety guidelines on alcohol use, simply search the internet for rules and regulations around consumption.

With respect to recreational drug use, there are no safety guidelines as to how much or how often they can be used or taken. There is the potential for great harm caused from a one-time, give-it-a-go event, or from multiple regular use. The potential for harm far outweighs the temporary numbness or euphoric feeling you may get from taking them.

Below is Hannah's story describing her drug use after an event involving sexual abuse. If this raises any concerns regarding sexual, physical or emotional abuse for you, I urge you to please reach out to a trustworthy adult who is empathetic and caring. By telling someone, it doesn't necessarily mean everything will change all at once, but it can mean you do not have to carry a heavy load all by yourself anymore.

It is really smart to tap into any resource available to you such as talking with your GP, doctor, psychologist, school counsellor or someone from a victim support helpline to make sure you and your situation are safe.

Hannah's story

I am not a victim. I am not somebody who needs saving; I am not a damsel in distress. However, I will forever be known by my friends, family and teachers as the girl who was sexually abused. I had decided the night it happened that I would keep my mouth shut, and I did, for 324 days. I kept this secret in my chest. Judge me if you want, call me stupid and naive, but I had my reasons.

For many months, a fire of rage burned within me affecting all parts of my life, but eventually it turned to a pile of extinguished ash. Without the adrenaline of seeking revenge or an apology I would never receive to fuel me, I became completely empty. I'm ashamed to admit that I turned to the easiest coping mechanism to ease my own trauma.

I used external substances to feel even the slightest bit of emotion. A high would only last three hours, and the comedown made me nauseous and cranky, but it was better than feeling nothing. Even though I knew it was wrong, that it was a path I never wanted to stumble down, I let myself do so anyway. Maybe it was self-pity and shame, but at least I knew I had a problem. I was a self-aware idiot. I know excuses can only validate my actions so far. But I can say I never let my angry, numb, drug-fuelled highs affect anyone around me. No one noticed me drowning. I think that's what made it worse. I had no shoulder to cry on, no support to hold me when my legs went wobbly. I was alone.

But in this dark lonely place, I found myself. Not the person I display to the world; rather I found my bare-boned soul. In my grief, I managed to find what most teenagers spend their whole high school life searching for. I had found myself. I built myself from the ground up. I nurtured my caring, broken soul and made it back to what it once was. In the silent, dark, numb place I had stumbled into somewhere in-between the raging fire and the quiet forest. I healed.

I began my healing journey by letting that coat of silence slip off my shoulders. Telling my friends and family was extremely hard and sometimes I almost regret telling them, but in the end, I knew I was on my way to healing. Yes, my scars still bleed and my eyes still water, but I have begun my journey to heal. I am not a victim; I am strong. I am not somebody who needed saving; I saved myself. I am not a damsel in distress; I am independent and worthy of my journey to heal.

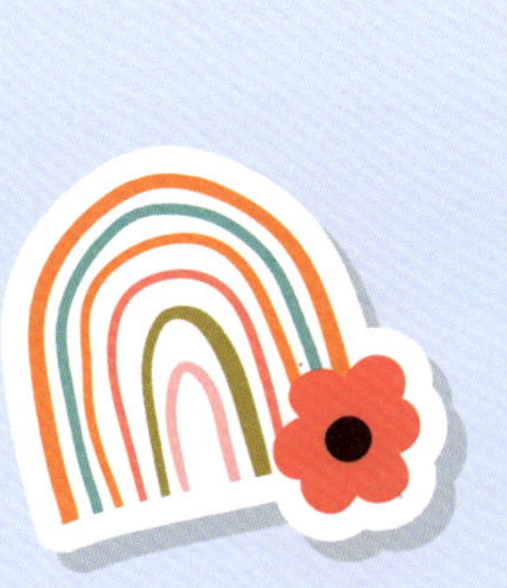

Some use food or self-harming as a way to manage their extremely overwhelming feelings.

Eating disorders are more than just about regulating food intake. They are a range of psychological conditions that lead to the development of unhealthy eating behaviours. Everyone has 'fat days' from overeating or maybe some odd eating habits. However, a true eating disorder involves the use of extreme excessive behaviours to control weight and body shape.

Fashionable body shape has been around for decades and decades, through what we saw in print and movies a hundred years ago through to what we see through social media today. Society as a whole imposes such unrealistic beauty standards and expectations with relentless pressure to look a certain way.

In the few short years of being a teenager, your body is flooded with hormones and growth spurts as you move from being a child to a young adult. A lot of physical change occurs in this time and most of it will be governed by your genetic makeup.

It is imperative to not compare yourself, your body shape or look to others, as some teens will be naturally tall and thin or medium and curvy or short and sporty. Some 'fill out' or grow tall before they even reach puberty, while, for others, it may take until their late teens. Your body will keep changing — please be patient with it.

As eating disorders can be precarious with good days and bad days, it's good to remind yourself what's at stake — your physical health and emotional wellbeing. A good way to combat the harder days is to ensure your emotional needs are being met.

Find something that gives you meaning or a purpose in your life. Anything that gives you something to look forward to, makes you feel good about yourself or provides a sense of achievement in your life. It can be easier to look after your nutritional needs once feeling more settled, content and good about yourself.

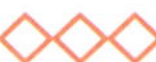

If you are self-harming, it is essential for you to please reach out to someone you trust, who is empathetic and caring. They do not need to have the ability to fix everything, but can be there for you in that moment, as *you deserve a compassionate and considerate response.*

As the moment passes, please keep opening up and talk with your family, GP, psychologist, school counsellor or someone from the various help lines available, so you may receive ongoing help and support. It is their job to talk about embarrassing, private or difficult stuff — they do it every day.

There are a numerous helplines available, from youth helplines, anxiety/depression helplines, victim support, lifeline, suicide crisis lines, and drug and alcohol helplines to rainbow youth lines. A Google search will give you a range of numbers to call.

In the upcoming pages are a variety of coping strategies you may like to try including healthy coping behaviours, tapping techniques and the power of forgiveness. First though, is Paige's story. It is a moving account of her journey with self-harming.

Paige's story

A couple of years ago I stopped self-harming and started managing my anxiety. I saw, and still see, the school counsellor and got a part-time job after school. I have learned that the best help has to come from me first. And that is not easy, as I still struggle with a lot of stuff.

I started self-harming when I began high school. I was thirteen. Looking back now, I couldn't tell you exactly why I started, what the catalyst was, I just think there was a lot going on and emotionally I did not know how to handle some people and situations. I do remember feeling quite disconnected with everything and everyone, and struggled with some of my friendships. I have had anxiety and panic attacks since I was young. I know people saw me as a happy child but I did not feel that way.

Self-harming was a horrible cycle of not coping well, wanting to harm, harming, then feeling pathetic and guilty afterwards. When people asked me about my cuts and scars, my thoughts were bombarded with 'What do I say?', 'They know I'm lying', 'I sound pathetic', but mostly, the main thought was, 'It's none of your business. This is my body, back off.'

I couldn't tell my family, even though I get on well with them, though eventually Mum saw the marks and we talked about it. She just listened with sympathy and no judgement.

She asked questions to help me express my feelings and, at the end of it, I felt relief that she knew. I was so scared she would feel bad about what I was doing and blame herself. I know other kids are scared their parents will get mad or judge them, or make it about themselves, that's why self-harming is usually hidden.

She didn't try to fix me — well, there was advice cos she's a mum and can't help herself. With my harming being more out in the open, and with Mum's support, I started to manage my feelings by doing things I like and, as I said, I see the school counsellor and got a part-time job, which makes me feel more independent and confident.

I try to do different things every day that make me happy. I like to listen to music, watch movies I love, paint and draw. I did gratitude and forgiveness techniques — they helped at the time. I got an app on my phone where I could record how long I did not self-harm and every day I logged in and wrote how I was feeling. I found that good, seeing how many days I didn't do it.

I've learned to try to take life one day at a time!

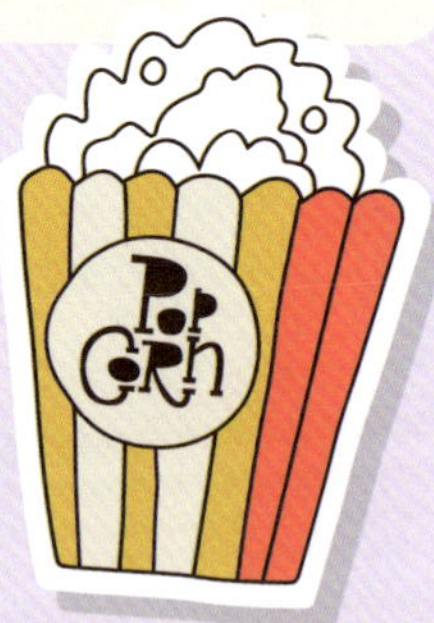

8.

Healthy Coping Habits

Here is a range of distraction methods for a variety of feelings you may like to try. You may need a couple of them, as no two experiences are ever exactly same.

When feeling fearful or sad, try:

- getting out in nature. Be aware of the trees, the sky, all your surroundings. Nature has high energy levels and we always feel better from being outside. It is soothing and uplifting
- putting on music you enjoy – uplifting tunes you can listen, sing or dance to
- a tapping technique (see Tapping Exercises on page 37) — for stress, fear or anxiety
- using a heavy blanket, which can be soothing, ensures a safe, comfortable feeling when wrapped around you. There are specifically designed blankets to improve sleep, reduce

stress and anxiety. Look at 'calming blanket' or 'therapy blanket'

- interacting with an animal. Play with or hug an animal, or take the dog for a walk
- talking with someone about how you are feeling.

When you are feeling shameful or guilty, remember:

- when you are being open, honest and conducting yourself with integrity, you are not responsible for other people's actions, feelings or words. Therefore, there is no need to feel regret, shame or guilt when you are being your authentic respectful self
- if you have said or acted in a way that has led you to feel this way, try the forgiveness techniques coming up on page 41
- to accept that making mistakes is part of being human — we all make them! They are simply an opportunity to learn and move on from
- stop spending time with people who do not treat you with respect, value your opinion or who are unkind to you.

When you feel everything is out of your control, try:

- tidying up your room or getting out into a garden and pulling out some weeds — make it look nice

- decluttering your bedroom or any other space you are allowed to
- writing lists of what needs to be done, prioritizing the tasks
- writing in a journal or on a piece of paper expressing your feelings. Being able to express how you feel is important; writing is just one way. You can even rip it up after
- to stop, pause and breathe in deeply, hold and then exhale slowly, maybe a few times. This is like hitting a reset button. It allows all those out-of-control, scattered thoughts to settle so you can become aware of the present moment, calming your nervous system and providing clarity and focus.

When feeling frustrated or angry, try:

- picking up a cushion and hitting the ground with it or shouting into it. Note: when expressing frustration or anger physically like this, it does not work for everyone. If this intensifies your feelings, try one of the below instead
- movement — use those inward angry feelings to fuel vigorous exercise like running, boxing or going to the gym
- ripping pieces of paper or fabric into hundreds of tiny pieces.

When feeling disconnected or numb, try:

- using movement to feel your heart rate, sweat and muscles. For some, emotional numbness feels like they are frozen, so movement can help
- holding ice cubes, moving them around in your hands
- smelling something with a very strong odour.

9.

Tapping Exercises

Several different therapies use the technique of 'tapping'. Energy Medicine and Emotional Freedom Technique (EFT) are two well-known ones. Tapping on various points on your body helps balance your energy and reduces emotional or physical pain. It sends a calming signal to your brain to relax, which slows the release of stress hormones, allowing you to feel better.

There are numerous tapping clips on YouTube and social media. My favourite clips are from Nick Ortner, but there are many others available.

Here is a selection of tapping techniques to get you started.

Start with gentle tapping for about 10–20 seconds or until it feels right to stop. Use one or two fingers from each hand.

The karate chop for all emotions

Use the tips of your fingers from one hand to gently tap the soft area on the side of the other hand, just below your little finger.

It's the part of your hand you would use if you were to 'karate chop' something. Tune into what you are feeling, such as stressed, anxious, angry, down, overwhelmed or in pain (physical or mental). Focus on what feelings you want to change or let go of and say these statements to yourself while tapping this area of your hand:

'Even though I have this ... [stress/anxiety/hurt — choose what is appropriate] in my body, I choose to relax now.'

'Even though I have all this ... stress [or other feeling] and it's hard to let go, I am open to releasing it now.'

'Even though I am holding on to all this ... stress [or other feeling], I choose to let it go now.'

Repeat as needed.

Specific tapping

Increase energy levels: tap the area about five centimetres / two inches below the middle of each collarbone, on both sides of your chest — it is the area on both sides of your thymus gland. This is called the K27 junction or point.

Grounding: Tap your cheeks just under the bony part of your cheek bones.

Reducing stress: Place your fingertips on your closed eyes, breathe in while pressing down and pull your fingertips towards your temples, continuing over and around your ears and down to the back of your shoulders. Then release the breath while running your fingertips from the back of your shoulders up and over to your heart. Repeat as needed.

Disrupting negative thoughts: First tap the K27 point to increase your energy (as above), then press a finger just above the middle of both eyebrows. You may continue to have the thoughts, but by holding these points, you make sure the upset doesn't have an adverse effect on your body or energy.

Anxiety tap: this is also known as the temporal tap. There is a structural line on the skull (your head) around the ears that, by tapping on it, while saying affirmations, has been found to directly connect to receptors related to anxiety. The right side of the head relates to negative statements and the left to positive. Tap firmly on your head around your ear. Start at your temple, tapping up, over and around behind your ear (you are tapping on your head around your ear, not on your ear).

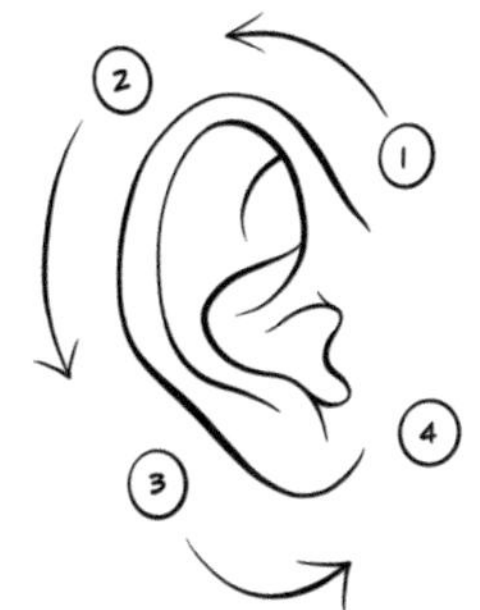

Say the affirmation as you tap. Start on the right ear, making a negative statement using words such as 'never', 'no' or 'not'. Then, on the left ear, make a positive statement using words such as 'I will' or 'I am'. For example, if you were worried about exams say this:

Right ear, tap and say, '*I am not* worried about my exams.' Repeat three times.

Left ear, tap and say, '*I will do* well in my exams.' Repeat three times.

Fear or phobias: Tap on your cheek bones under your eyes, in the rhythm of a waltz (1, 2, 3 ... 1, 2, 3). This connects to the receptors that deal with fear. Tap while firmly saying, 'I have no fear of ...'. You can do this for general fear, like fear of your future. When faced with a specific fear, such as a fear of heights, tap while you are standing somewhere up high (assuming it is safe to do so and you don't need to use both hands to hold on!).

Increasing Self-Esteem: Lack of self-esteem is often the main cause of anxiety and feeling overwhelmed and low, as we are extremely good at putting ourselves down and not so good at recognising our true self-worth. Tap on your thymus gland, as it is connected to your self-esteem. It is situated just below where your clavicle (collar) bones meet in the middle of your upper chest area. By tapping the thymus and thinking good things about yourself, it restores your self-esteem and enhances your health.

10.

Forgiveness

'Forgiveness does not change the past, but it does enlarge the future.'

—PAUL BOESE

Forgiveness is a good practice for releasing painful emotions or any feelings tied to a past event that stops us from moving forward. Forgiveness benefits the forgiver; it is the gift we give ourselves, as when we do, it starts the process of improving our life circumstances.

It starts with forgiving ourselves for any past wrongdoings or decisions, then forgiving others for their wrongdoings, words or actions that have hurt us. You can even forgive injustices in life in general.

The mistakes we make do not make us a bad person and, yes, we still deserve to live a happy life. Everyone messes up — learning to forgive ourselves, let go and move on is a wonderful tool as it helps us let go of shame, guilt, frustration and sadness. If we do not learn how to, as 'like attracts like', we run the risk of attracting more of the same back to us.

'Forgiveness does not mean accepting the wrongdoing of the other person, but to retain a feeling of anger, hatred or stress does more harm to yourself than the actual act of forgiving.

The real meaning of forgiveness is to mentally not develop feelings of anger and hatred due to the wrong actions of others.'

—DALAI LAMA

When forgiving someone else, it does not mean we have to welcome them back into our life or become their best friend again; rather, it releases us from continually holding any hurt, anger, bitterness or resentment caused by their hurtful words or actions. Staying hurt and resentful towards them is a bit like picking up a hot piece of coal to throw at them. This process only burns ourselves.

'You can forgive some people without welcoming them back into your life. Apology accepted; access denied.'

—@POWER OF POSITIVITY

When forgiving someone, you do not have to forgive them to their face. The words of forgiveness can be said out loud or written in a letter that does not get sent.

Either way, your subconscious mind hears the message of forgiveness. It does not know if the person is right in front of you or not. It cannot see or analyse; it simply hears and records the words of forgiveness, allowing it to shift any limiting or negative perception around the feelings towards the person or situation.

It may have to be said or read several times before actually feeling the shift in your perception — this is okay. Or you may simply just choose: 'Right here, right now, I choose not to hold these feelings of injustice anymore, I'm free to get on with my life.'

Forgiveness provides the opportunity to release these negative emotions, which in turn creates space for new opportunities. You could then use an affirmation to fill that space with positive beliefs and thoughts. See Affirmations on page 14.

If you struggle to forgive yourself or someone else, here are some options you could consider.

Affirmations

'I am willing to forgive those who I perceive have hurt me in my past. I do so with love and non-judgement.'

'I forgive myself for any known or unknown mistakes I have made; I do so with love and non-judgement.'

'I forgive myself for believing I have to hold anger when I am bullied.'

'I forgive myself for believing it is my fault when I am bullied.'

Forgiveness exercise

Choose the person or situation you wish to forgive.

Note three things you gained from the relationship or situation. There is always something to be learned from every situation.

Write down what could have been happening in their life that you may not have known about, something that led to them to behave in a hurtful manner. For example, add a back story about them that helps you forgive their actions or words. It may be true or not. This is okay as it is just a tool to help you forgive and move forward. The aim is to help you see the situation from a new perspective. For example, you could write that you know they were lashing out and being mean, as their partner had just dumped them.

Next, visualize the person and situation and see yourself with them saying the following:

> 'May you (name) be happy, live in peace and know love.'
>
> 'May I be happy, live in peace and know love.'
>
> 'May we be happy, live in peace and know love.'

**'When we forgive, we heal.
When we let go, we grow.'**

—UNKNOWN

Here is an example of a letter written by Lily to help her move forward after her boyfriend cheated on her, and the wisdom and strength she gained through the process of forgiveness.

Lily's story

I am seventeen years old. I wrote this letter to express what it felt like going through the process of getting cheated on and how I have learned to not let it control my life or emotions anymore, as well as how the experience has allowed me to learn more about myself and become a better person:

From the moment I first met you I knew you were going to have an influence on my life, but just not in the ways you did. You taught me many things I am now able to look back on and appreciate, as each obstacle you threw in my direction has allowed me to be the person I am today. I am stronger because of you. I am kinder because of you. I am more forgiving and accepting because of you.

This letter is to allow me to have closure and express any last grieving emotions I have towards our relationship. I want to allow myself to be free of you. Free from the resentment I have towards you and your actions. I want to break free from the chokehold your actions have on my emotions. Although the scars your infidelity caused may never fade completely, I refuse to let them define me. I no longer want to be a person who experiences any bitterness and displeasure towards actions I had no control over. I know that by doing so, the past will no longer continue to impact my present.

I would like to begin by saying thank you. I will never regret being with you, as our relationship provided both of us with a connection we had never experienced before. At the end of the day we both tried our best.

What you did to me, though, made me feel worthless and foolish. The first time it happened, for months it felt like my heart had been ripped out of my chest and torn to pieces right in front of me. I will never forget her name or the way her long honey-brown hair draped over your shoulders as you pushed her hair out of her face. For a long time, I blamed myself. Over time, I have accepted that your actions were not my doing and have let go of any feelings that I could have changed the narrative of our story ending.

The second time you betrayed me, despite being at a festival with thousands of people, I felt alone. My internal thoughts were, 'It happened again. It has to be my fault; there must be something wrong with me.' Maybe I was not good enough? Without the reassurance of my parents' words and hugs, I was left battling these notions myself. Although I would have done anything to not be at the festival surrounded by the constant reminder of what you did, I believe I am stronger as I became my own comfort person. You helped me realise I only need myself and anyone else I have in my life is an added bonus. I am now a better person because of it.

Thank you for the memories we shared. Despite how we ended, I am thankful for the many moments of joy and pure happiness throughout our relationship. You have taught me valuable lessons, which posed as stepping stones in the pathway towards my personal growth. Thank you for allowing me to create a better version of myself that you will never get to experience.

Life is far too short for either of us to retain ill feelings. I truly hope we can both move forward in a positive approach. May we both find happiness on our individual paths. I wish you all the best.

Lily.

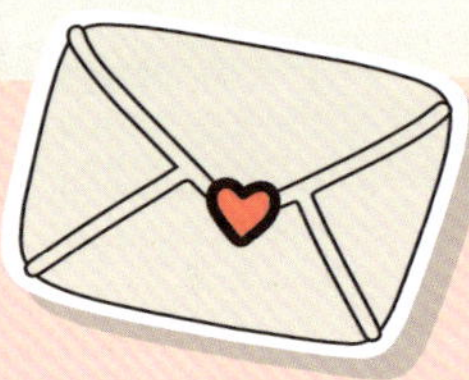

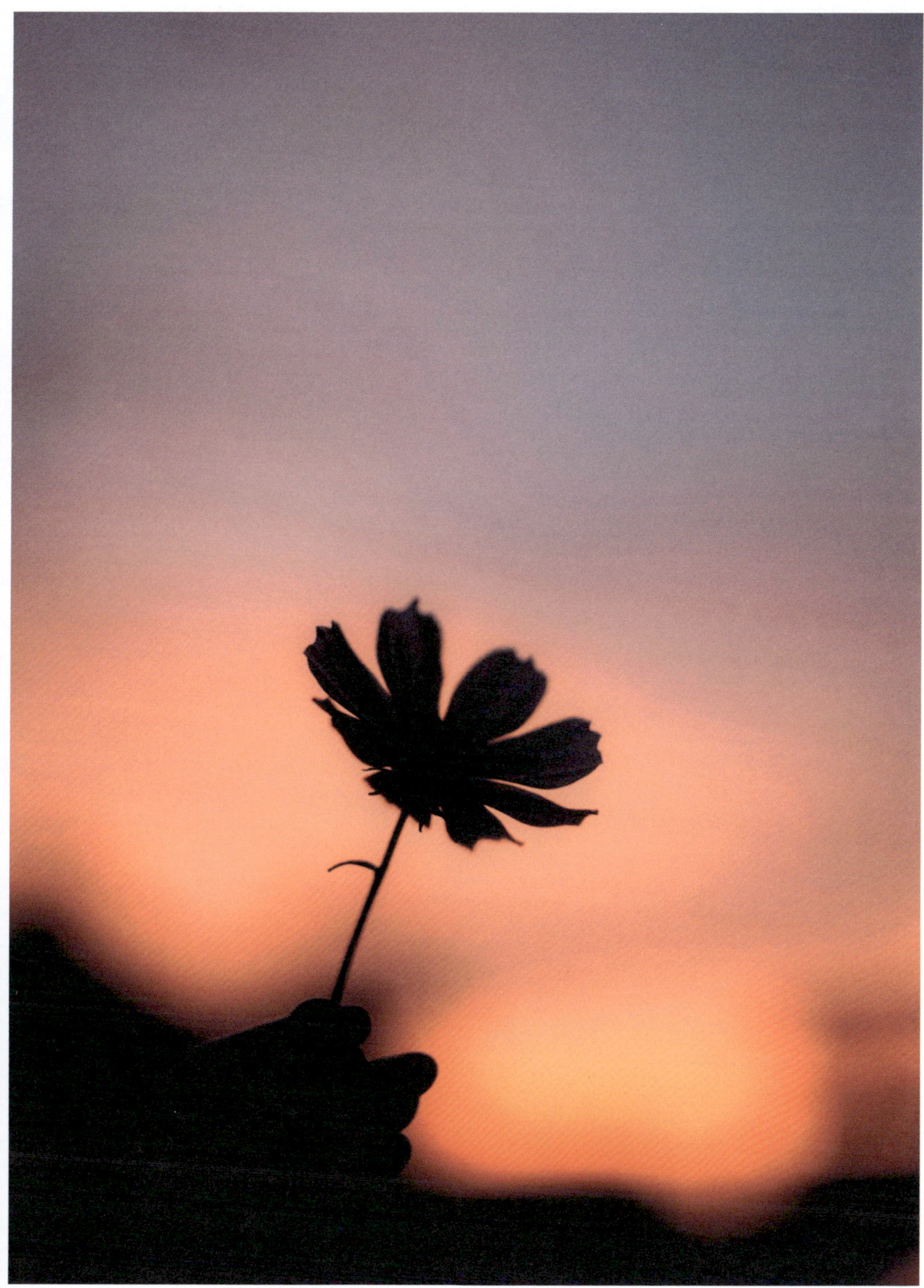

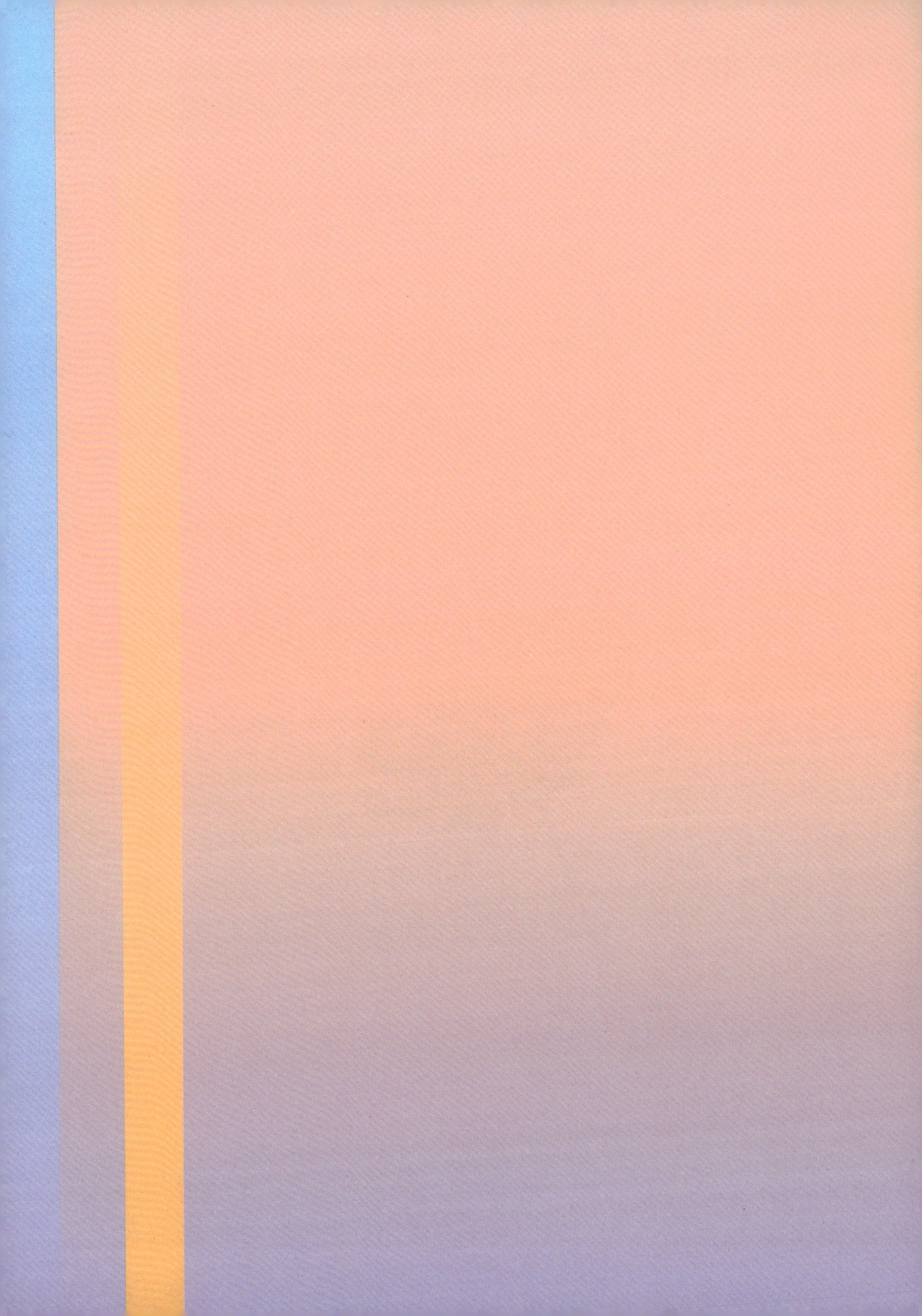

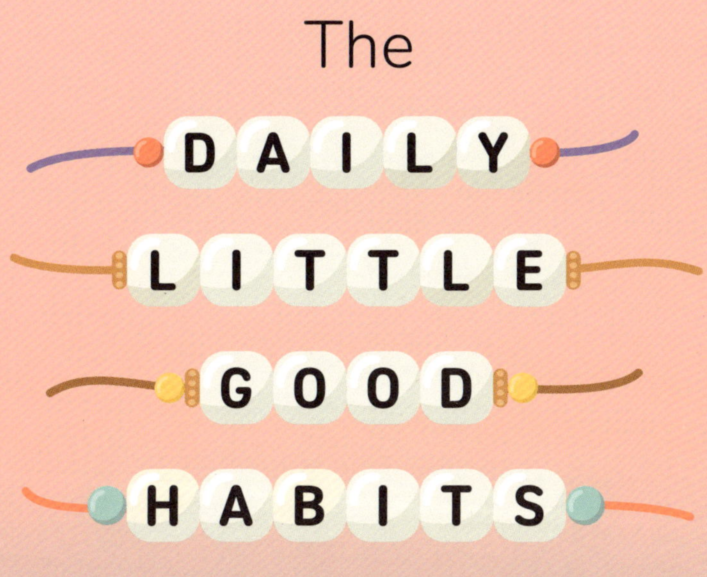

Toolkit

11.

Fight, Flight, Freeze or Please

Stress, worry and sadness are all a normal part of being human, as is fear — in fact, they can be essential for our survival. However, these feelings can have a negative impact on our wellbeing. If left too long without managing them, they will trigger our fight or flight (stress) response.

This response is controlled by our nervous system and kicks in when we feel threatened, overwhelmed, stressed, worried or have feelings of despair. It releases a variety of stress hormones, such as adrenaline and cortisol, to help us face danger and deal with the things making us feel this way.

Adrenaline increases blood flow to our heart, limbs and muscles in case we need to fight or flee the perceived danger. This often causes our heart to race, making it difficult to breathe. For some, this brings on a panic attack.

Cortisol creates fear to make us act, to deal with the stress or trigger. This can fuel negative thoughts because of its role in helping us face danger.

When we are in fight or flight mode, the brain dampens down our digestive function as it is not immediately needed when trying to cope with the stress. The issue with this is our gut contains most of our immune cells that keep us well and nervous system cells that make important neurotransmitters that lift our mood, like serotonin and dopamine.

Serotonin helps regulate our mood as it is responsible for our emotions, in particular our happiness.

Dopamine is responsible for allowing us to feel pleasure, motivated and satisfied.

Therefore, in stressful situations, or when we feel anxious, down or scared and so on, our body increases the number of stress hormones that stimulate our negative thoughts to make us act to fix the problem and gets our heart pumping, preparing to fight or flee — at the same time, it cannot make the happier chemicals to counteract them. It's a double whammy of bad news.

Typical symptoms of when our body is in fight or flight mode are heart palpitations; jitteriness; a feeling of being out of balance, uneven or like we're walking through quicksand or on a tight rope; a variety of gut dysfunction issues like IBS, constipation or diarrhoea; sleep dysfunction and insomnia; poor immunity with repeated colds or taking a long time to recover from illnesses;

fatigue; brain fog; poor concentration and memory; and anxiety, panic attacks and mild depression.

On the positive side, we can do a variety of things each day to help increase our serotonin levels naturally and reduce our cortisol levels by switching off our fight or flight response and relaxing.

One easy thing to do when the adrenaline is pumping around the body is to literally shake it off — make your body shake, do some star jumps, dance — anything with vigorous movement to use up that adrenaline.

A little sensory stimulation increases our serotonin levels when we listen, touch, smell or taste something that calms our nervous system. For example:

Use essential oils. Choose one that has a calming effect on the nervous system. For example, lavender is the most well-known oil to soothe and relax, helping reduce anxiety and promote sleep; frankincense has been used for centuries to increase relaxation and reduce stress; and bergamot also reduces stress and enhances our mood.

Specific sound frequencies are known to calm. 639 Hz tackles negative feelings and heals the heart and 852 Hz helps relieve tension and promotes better sleep. You can find a variety of music with specific Hz frequencies on YouTube and the internet. Or just have calming music playing in the background.

Touch various shapes and textures. For example, rub a fluffy pillow (or an animal) or play with a sequined garment, rubbing back and forth as it changes colour or shape.

To help relax and switch off your fight or flight mode, start one or two of these stimulation activities daily, as little good habits of wellness. They work by bringing your focus to the present moment. Not in the past where guilt, shame, regret or sadness reside, nor the future, where fear and anxiety reside. These daily habits help embed positive changes in our lives, improving our thoughts and feelings.

Never underestimate the power of small habits! If you were to read ten pages a day, you would have read fifteen or more books a year, or if you save $6 per day, that would give you $2,190 at the end of the year.

Simply put, daily habits of wellbeing increase happy hormones and reduce stress hormones: ergo, better mental health.

Take a look at some of the daily habit suggestions in the following sections. If done consistently, they create a foundation of good mental health. Pick the ones that gel with you so you are more likely to stick with them.

12.

Quiet Time

The magic of being still and quiet has a positive effect on our mental and emotional health as it automatically calms the nervous system. When and where you can, take a five-to-ten-minute mental break. Find a peaceful spot away from loud noises and people, where you can just sit quietly without any interruptions.

This can be the best remedy when you find yourself feeling overwhelmed and need time to untangle challenging situations. The intention is to allow yourself a moment to step back from all the emotions and frustrations. The mind will start to calm as the thoughts that come with those feelings recede, so when you go back to whatever you were doing, you can do so in a calmer, clearer way.

You can also use this time to reflect on your day. Are there things you are proud of? If so, acknowledge them.

It is often in our quiet moments that we have those 'a-ha' moments, when things seem to just fall into place and make sense, or clarity on a situation comes to light. We don't seem to get them when we're rushing around, as we are too busy to notice.

13.

Set Clear Intentions

How you spend the first 30 minutes of your day determines the trajectory for the rest of it. Starting it calmly and positively sets up the best intention for the day.

Try setting your alarm clock to wake up a little earlier each morning. In those few minutes before you get out of bed, set a clear intention for the day. Think about who you want to be and how you want to feel throughout the day. Visualize, sense and/or feel what that would be like.

If you have any tasks planned that day, visualize them being easily and successfully completed.

Taking the time to set clear, positive thoughts, feelings and intentions before getting out of bed gives you a great springboard to launch your day from. It may not stop the speed bumps from coming your way, but it can help you to handle them with more ease and clarity.

14.

Meditation

'Meditation is simply getting to know your mind.'

—DZOGCHEN PONLOP RINPOCHE

Daily meditations have proven to have many health benefits, including lowering stress levels and helping with sleep. They are a great way to quieten the mind. You can listen to a guided meditation to help you feel calm during the day or before going to sleep, or try just sitting quietly in a peaceful space while closing your eyes and focusing on your breathing.

There are many apps available. One I like is Insight Timer — it has hundreds of meditations on assisting with stress levels, anxiety and sleep, and loads of other topics. Other apps you could also try are Calm, Harmony or Headspace.

Meditation steps

To meditate you might like to sit in a comfortable chair with your back straight, feet flat on the floor, your hands resting in your lap, with your eyes closed. You could also sit on the ground, lean up against a wall or, alternatively, lie down.

Now the hard part — stopping those thoughts from racing through your mind! For most people, when first trying to meditate, this is the hardest part. It is very rarely instantly wonderful, and you will probably find yourself thinking you haven't got a clue what you are doing or that you are not very good at it. This is normal and, like most things, it takes practice — learning from mistakes and refining your techniques — until you're able do it more to your liking. Remember, your mind will never be completely blank. Therefore, it is about learning to let go of the distractions, allowing your mind to become calm and quieter.

Here are some points to follow:

Outside noise will always occur. Instead of trying to push away noises or let them annoy you, just accept them and let them be there; let them be part of the meditation. If you try to block them out, you will only hold onto them tighter, so just let them be.

Focus on your breathing. Take a long, slow breath in through your nose, hold for a moment, then blow it out through your nose or mouth on a long, slow exhale. Do this several times until you feel yourself relaxing. Let your shoulders relax as well as the muscles around your eyes, jaw, hips and legs. Feel the pull of gravity down into your core. Then allow your breathing to become soft, falling into a gentle, repetitive rhythm.

If a thought comes in, acknowledge it, then let it go. Use your out breath to gently nudge it away or visualize putting it in a bubble and seeing it float away. Know that if it is important, you will remember it afterwards.

Just try to experience the meditation in the moment rather than having any expectations; if those expectations are not met, it may lead to feelings of disappointment. Accept what you are able to do — your best in this moment — and enjoy the experience of the quietened mind. It's all about practice, practice, practice. Ideally, daily meditations are great, even if for five minutes. You can then build up to longer periods with practice when time allows.

15.

Step Outside

'Nature itself is the best physician.'

—HIPPOCRATES

Getting outside into nature, whether it's a stroll through a city park, or hiking up a mountain, generates positive emotions such as joy and peace. It has been linked to a range of health benefits, including improving our mood and concentration and reducing stress levels, which restores good mental health.

All nature has a high amount of energy that we naturally tap into, whether we know it or not — we always feel better and more energized from being outside in the fresh air. When we have higher energy levels, we become more resilient to life's ups and downs. Having low energy makes all tasks seem that much harder, generating more stress and worry. So, getting outside as much as possible can really help ... and it's free!

Take the dog for a walk or just yourself, take a dip at the beach, sit under a tree or up on a hill, relax in your garden or on your deck. Exercising outside has the dual benefits of sun exposure, making vitamin D and generating endorphins, both of which can help lift your mood. Gentle exercise may give you the space to feel present, but if you prefer it to be more vigorous, go for it!

If you are struggling with all the overwhelming bad news about our world that is being constantly streamed through news and social media platforms, then get out into nature. Nature reminds us how incredible our planet is.

16.

Mindfulness

'It is not that mindfulness is the "answer" to all life's problems. Rather, it is that all life's problems can be seen more clearly through a clear mind.'

—JON KABAT-ZINN

Being mindful means we are thinking, feeling and acting consciously, bringing us into the present moment. Being conscious and aware 24/7 is impossible, but we can build in times throughout our day to be mindful and present.

We can focus on our breathing (slowly in and out); eat mindfully (aware of each mouthful, enjoying the flavours); exercise mindfully (feeling our body respond); and have mindful posture (the way our body reflects confidence or unease). It can be like a type of meditation in which we focus on being aware of what we're sensing and feeling in the moment, without interpretation or judgement.

Sitting quietly, focusing on your *breathing* is like a form of meditation as mentioned earlier. Taking a deep breath in, holding it and then slowly exhaling is like a reset button for our nerves and the long exhale also calms the nervous system. As you exhale, relax any tension in your muscles and notice your shoulders dropping.

Keep observing your breath until any tension, anxiety or feelings of being overwhelmed start to fade.

You can also breathe calmly while thinking something positive like 'just breathe' or 'I am safe', as this brings your breathing and thoughts into alignment, making it faster for the mind and body to relax.

Another mindful act is to be *aware of each mouthful of food* as you eat, noting the texture and taking time to enjoy the flavours. As your thoughts focus on the present situation of eating, they are not scattered in other directions, allowing a sense of calmness. When finished, notice any foods that leave you feeling tired, lethargic or uncomfortable afterwards, as they are not lifting your vitality or energy or contributing to your health. They may be different for everyone and may take between 20 minutes to a couple of hours to occur. See more details in The Dietary Toolkit section.

To *exercise mindfully* means being aware of your environment, taking in the scenery. Looking up and about, what do you smell, hear, feel and see? Notice your footsteps, feel the ground and note any sun, wind or rain on your face. Again, this brings your focus to the present moment, allowing your feelings and thoughts to calm and clear as you notice and appreciate your environment.

Lastly, be *mindful of your posture.* Our body language is not only a signal to others of how we are feeling, but it is also a signal to our own brain, reinforcing how we are feeling. For example, when we feel frustrated, often our hands are clenched tightly together. Unclenching them lets some of the frustration lessen. When we feel sad our posture naturally slumps forward, like we are rolling into ourselves (it's a subconscious form of protection) and our eyebrows come together, creating a frown when we worry. All these postures alert our brain that something is not feeling right, just as much as our thoughts do.

Relaxing the muscles in your face, shoulders, hands, or anywhere where there is tension in the body, helps signal the brain to also relax.

17.

Gratitude

'As we express our gratitude, we must never forget that the highest appreciation is not to utter words, but to live by them.'

—JOHN F. KENNEDY

Have you noticed how all the things that make life worth living usually involve less thinking and more feeling? Feelings such as gratitude? Practising gratefulness is a really easy way to enhance our life. It takes us away from anxiety, greed, jealousy, taking things for granted and feelings of inadequacy or entitlement, and more towards appreciation, acceptance, contentment, joy and satisfaction.

These feelings lead to decreased levels of stress hormones and increased levels of happy hormones in the body, resulting in a reduction of anxious and sad thoughts and an improvement in mood.

Regardless of our life circumstances, the practice of consistent gratitude can be surprisingly difficult. It is easy to get caught up in bad news, unpleasant experiences and negative thoughts, yet allow those moments of positivity to fade quickly into the background. For instance, we may be so busy focusing on a verbal slip-up at a party that we do not register a compliment from a friend.

Adding to that, if we have a mental health concern, being able to see positive factors or express gratitude can seem unimaginable.

Luckily, gratitude is like a muscle you can build. Even in the hardest days, there is always something small to appreciate. Cultivating gratitude may seem silly but research has shown there are real health benefits from doing this practice, such as improving self-esteem, uplifting our mood and building stronger, healthier relationships.

How to practise gratitude

To practise gratitude, simply pick three things you are grateful for. They can be simple things, from having a nice hot chocolate to something you really love. The secret is to then reflect on *why* it was nice and deserves your gratitude and/or love. It's the describing or thinking of the 'why' that allows the feelings of gratitude to flow through you. As you remember, your positive feelings come into the present moment too, allowing a sense of connection to yourself and environment with more peace and contentment.

If you did the above before going to sleep, it will help shift you from mulling over the things you may feel anxious or down about, to the things you feel good about and, hopefully, this eases your mind so you may drift off to sleep, though it can be done at any time you want to shift negative feelings.

If you find yourself in a tough spot, start counting the things working for you or that are in your favour. They could be anything from having a roof over your head at night, that you had breakfast that morning, that you're good at study or have the ability to exercise. Those tough spots provide us with the opportunity to recognise the good things in our lives and be grateful for them.

Find things that inspire you, reminding you that life is beautiful. Spend time with people who demonstrate kindness, laughter and honesty; watch shows or documentaries that have heroic, honourable, loving, genuine people in them; or read inspiring novels or inspirational quotes. All these things encourage feelings of gratitude.

Daily gratitude is like medicine for the heart and soul, allowing happiness and wellbeing that can transform our lives.

18.

Get Grounded

Being grounded means we have a clear sense of who we are and how we are feeling in the present moment, as well as having a strong connection between ourselves and our environment. This allows us to be physically, mentally and emotionally sure of ourselves.

It provides us with mental clarity and focus, along with feeling purposeful. When we are too busy, rushed or thinking of the past or future, we lose awareness of what is real for us right now, which may intensify poor mental health.

Being grounded helps against those challenging times, to be more resilient and confident.

Doing daily, good habits of wellness, that make you pause and bring your awareness into the present moment, will ground you. However, here are some specific tips on how to feel grounded:

Walk outside on the grass, sand, dirt or in the shallow waters of an ocean, lake or river, where it is safe to do so. Anywhere outside is great and, if you can, go barefoot. Bring your attention to your feet and the connection between you and the ground, to really feel your presence on the earth.

Be still for a few minutes, allowing your uninterrupted focus to remain on that connection, being one with nature. As you breathe out, let your concerns fall away to the ground and, as you breathe in, let the earth's vibrant energy fill you up.

If you are unable to get outside, sit in a quiet place and listen to nature sounds through a device while imagining you are sitting in your favourite outdoor place. Close your eyes and feel the connection with nature and the earth. Again, breathe out worries and breathe in the earth's energy.

If connecting with nature is not really your thing, or you are somewhere where it is hard to do, this grounding exercise may suit you better. It is particularly good to do when feeling overwhelmed or if a panic attack is coming on:

To bring you back to the present moment, right now, in your mind ...

- List five things you can see. Note them in detail.
- Name four things you can physically feel.
- Listen for three things you can hear, including distant sounds.
- Note two things you can smell.
- Name one thing you can taste OR one thing you are grateful for.

19.

A Dose of Laughter

**'Always laugh when you can.
It is cheap medicine.'**

—LORD BYRON

We all need to laugh more and find ways to lighten our mood and not take everything so seriously.

To do this, think about what brings you joy. What activities do you like doing? You may have a few. If you can do one or more of them every day, it helps balance out the challenging moments when they arise.

When you feel low, watch funny YouTube or TikTok clips, a comedy movie, something that makes you laugh, as this will naturally shift and lift your energy.

It's easier to release those daily worries and stressors when you are laughing, as it gets those happy hormones humming. To help lighten a dark mood, listen, sing and dance to your favourite tunes, get a hug from someone you love, play with an animal and put things around you that make you feel happy.

It is not about trying to be happy 24/7 — that could lead to the mask slipping on: looking happy, feeling crappy. Rather, it helps us to lighten up and reminds us not to take life so seriously. It helps to bring balance into our lives, between those bad and good moments. When the laughter fades and the challenges return, it gives us a chance to look at them through a lighter heart with a happier filter. These moments of laughter provide a mental break our mind often needs, even if just for a little while.

Never feel bad or guilty for feeling happy or laughing. Be the inspirations for others to be and do the same. The more people can laugh, the better and lighter life can become.

20.

Journalling

'I can shake off everything as I write; my sorrows disappear, my courage is reborn.'

—ANNE FRANK

Journalling is a great exercise to express any emotions that have been bottled up inside, or to simply write about your day. Doodle, write songs, poems, affirmations or just what you are grateful for — these are also examples of journalling. Basically, anything you want to get off your chest or feel inspired to convey in the moment.

The intent of expressing emotions through pen and paper is to take any anguish inside you and physically put it outside you onto the paper. This starts the process of releasing and letting go of discouraging thoughts and feelings.

You do not have to keep it. You can rip it up, bury or burn it if that feels right to do so. You could even make this into a little ceremony if that helps to let the feelings go.

Before you do, though, it can be interesting to read what you wrote, as it is possible to be unaware of what's really on your mind until you read it!

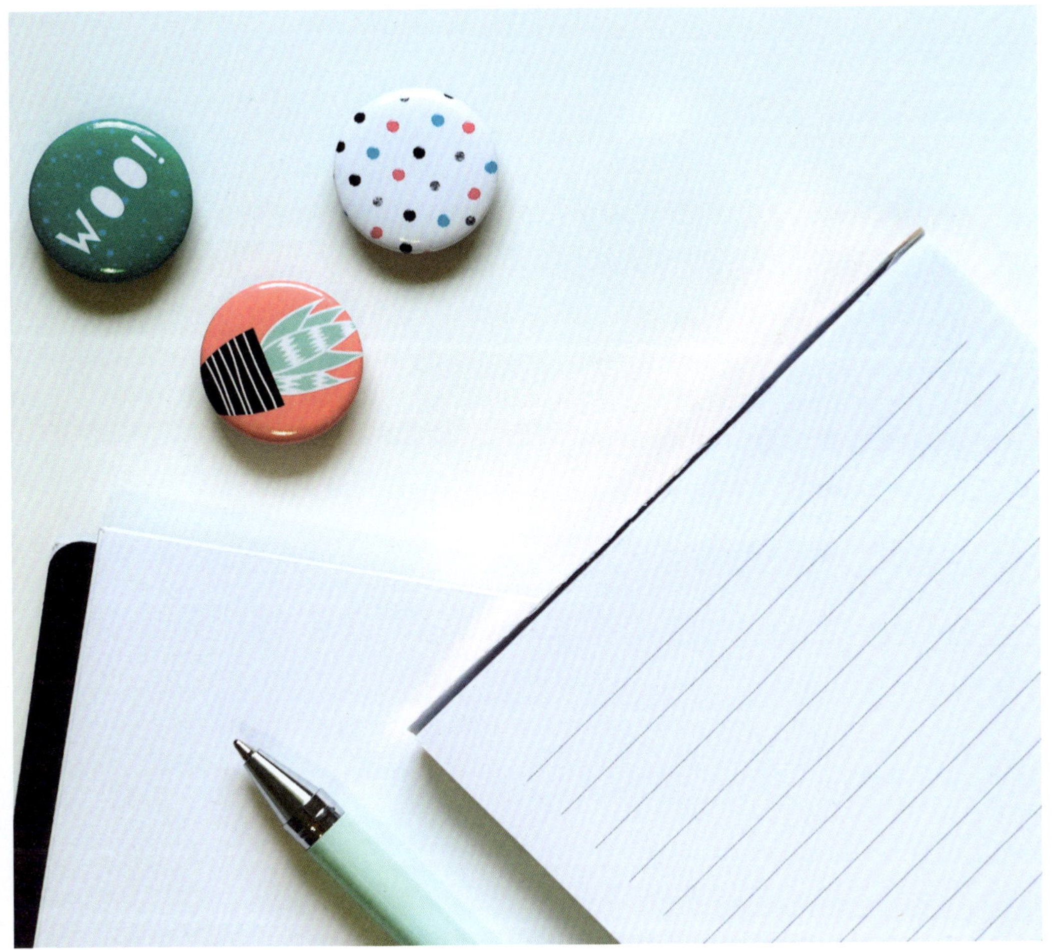

The ENERGETIC VIBES Toolkit

21.

Manifesting

We become what we think about. Energy flows where your attention goes.'

—RHONDA BYRNE

There are four attributes that make you human: your physical, mental, emotional and energy aspects. All these make you YOU.

Think of yourself as a four-legged chair. Each leg represents your four aspects. If one leg is unwell, broken or ignored, its function diminishes.

This will ultimately affect the function of the whole — being a chair to easily sit upon.

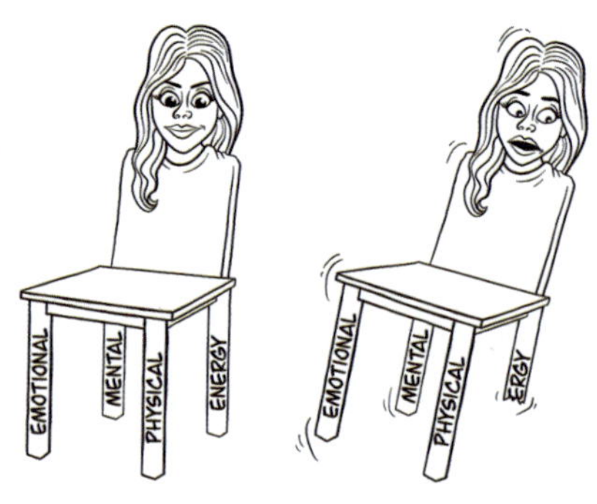

Your four aspects do not work in isolation — they work together, just like the four legs of the chair do.

This means you can use your energy to positively affect the other three aspects and your life experiences.

Our thoughts, words, cells and inner being are all energy and together they make our unique energetic frequency or vibe. Our energy is part of a sea of energy that makes up the whole cosmos, as energy is everywhere and in everything, and it can interact with this sea of energy. For example, have you ever been thinking of someone, then they call and you hear yourself saying, 'I was just thinking about you'? That's energy interacting within our environment and with us.

All energy has the ability to attract or repel other energies. Think of it as magnetic. Our energy can attract and cling to other energy frequencies that are similar to our own, attracting similar people or situations to us. Or our energy can repel those with different frequencies that are not like us.

This is how the law of attraction and manifesting work, as *energies that vibrate at the same frequency are attracted to one another.* So, to manifest or attract something positive into our lives, we need our energetic vibes to match the thing we wish for.

For example, if we want to attract a new best friend into our life, but deep down we feel or believe we are not good enough, our vibrational wish is not matching our vibrational feelings and beliefs. When the energy contained within our beliefs, thoughts, feelings and desires are in line with one another, the energy of intention will be clear and strong to start attracting the new friend. Then we need to act, to actually get out there with our clear, aligned intentions to find them.

Unfortunately, this also works in the same way when we have negative thoughts and feelings. If we are feeling overwhelmed, depressed or anxious, we will think and act upon those undesirable feelings and this will attract more of the same back to us, and repel the happier ones away.

Picture for a moment a person who is depressed and the vibes they give off. Then picture someone who is really happy or in love, and the vibes they give off. You can see, feel and sense the different vibes.

> **'Everything is energy and that's all there is to it. Match the frequency of the reality you want and you cannot help but get that reality. It can be no other way. This is not philosophy, this is physics.'**
>
> —ALBERT EINSTEIN

In other words, this is not woo woo. This is science!

> **To attract or manifest something in to our life, we have to feel, believe and act *right now* like we already have it.**

This brings our energy in line with the energy of what we are trying to attract. If for example, we want to attract more love, then we have to *feel, believe and act* lovingly towards ourselves and to the people within our community now. If we want more success, then we have to feel, believe and act successful right now, and so on.

An easy way to do this is to picture yourself as having achieved the goal or living your dream life, and note how that feels. For instance, would it make you feel free, happy, content? Then bring those specific feelings of freedom, happiness and contentment, or whatever they may be, to your present moment as often as possible. Take a few seconds, several times throughout your day, to stop and picture yourself living your dreams and allow those positive feelings to fill you up and shift your energy to that same vibration. Then let your thoughts and actions follow suit.

> **What's inside you, your thoughts and emotions, coupled with your actions, is what you will attract more of.**

There are specific manifesting and abundance meditations you can listen to that align your energy with your beliefs and feelings. One of my favourites is on the Insight Timer App, though a variety can be found on the internet and YouTube.

The best time to listen to one is upon waking for five to ten minutes every day, or as you drift off to sleep, as your brain waves are in theta state (the time between sleep and wakefulness) and the messages go straight into the subconscious mind. You can of course listen to them at any time if that suits you better.

Using affirmations discussed earlier on page 14 can also help do this, as they help align the energy of our beliefs to the energy of our desires.

Likewise, it is the same principal as the Placebo Effect, mentioned earlier on page 20, as believing, thinking and acting positively allows us to be the chemist of our own blood, manifesting and directing our mental and emotional wellbeing for the better.

When you start manifesting something, there can be things standing in the way of you achieving your desired outcome. Some things may have to end for better things to begin. For instance, say you want to manifest more money. The journey to receiving that money might require you to first lose your job in order to be free to accept a better-paid job.

When manifesting, remember, things will start to shift and change. This may not necessarily happen all at once — it might be a little each day or every few days. Also, it may not be what you had in mind or expected, but please stay patient and stick with it — while the journey to your ultimate goal may not be what you pictured, it could lead to something even better than you imagined.

22.

Trust Your Vibes

**'In science we call it energy.
In religion we call it spirit.
In the streets we call it vibes.
All I'm saying is trust it!'**

—@POWER OF POSITIVITY

Energy carries intelligence and is full of knowledge. It can interact and communicate through space, through the sea of energy that is everywhere. Our ability to interact with or tune into this sea and understand it is often referred to as our intuition.

Our intuitive instinct stems from and through our energy being, which can be thought of as being our inner voice of wisdom.

So, what exactly is intuition? It is the ability to understand something instinctively without the need for conscious reasoning or thinking. It helps us to understand and overcome stress, worries or doubts when we listen and act upon it.

Intuitive thoughts and feelings are not things we analyse or ponder on — that's our mind. Rather, they arise rapidly, seemingly out of nowhere. Please know, your intuitive instinct knows what is best for you even if your mind is taking a while to get with the programme.

> **It is so important to trust and act upon your instinct. Its number one priority is to protect you — always!**

Learning to listen and act upon your instincts can keep you safe. For example, if something feels 'off' or makes you feel uncomfortable, *leave*. When hopping into a car, if you doubt the driver, *don't get in*.

> **It is more important to listen to your instinct than it is to your friends or peers.**

Those instincts also help to achieve a happy balance between your thoughts, feelings and actions if you are willing to be open and honest with yourself. It is the alignment between your integrity and being authentic — being true to yourself.

Your integrity guides you to do what is right and what is for the best. This makes it directly connected with your intuition, as they do the same thing, working together.

Both provide a sense of purpose and direction, like a compass ensuring you do what feels right to keep yourself safe and happy. When you act with integrity it is important to remember that, whatever you say or do, you do so with the best intention (with honesty), regardless of the outcome. It does not matter what anyone else thinks, it only matters what you think and feel.

Consider that compass as uniting your Mind–Body–Soul connection. This connection is natural and contains intuitive knowledge about what is right for you and what you need to be emotionally, mentally and physically healthy.

There are lots of ways to access and use your intuition. It comes through all your senses — what you see, hear, feel, smell, taste — and those instincts of just 'knowing' stuff. The trick is to be aware of your own vibes, listen to them, trust them and then act accordingly.

It is often referred to as 'the little voice inside my head'. This intuitive guidance can be heard as if it were one of your own thoughts, but it's brief, to the point, not analysing or prattling on, and is often wise. As everyone has thousands of thoughts each day, sometimes those intuitive ones get lost among them; however, they are there and you may experience those 'a-ha' or 'what a coincidence' moments.

If you are unsure whether you have received intuitive guidance, check how it makes you feel. Intuitive guidance *always feels right* within you, like it sits well somewhere deep inside.

Sometimes we ignore our intuition, as it may be telling us something we are not ready to hear or do, or it involves having to make a difficult choice. Change can create anxiety. There is a difference, though, between intuitive guidance that may feel worrying than say everyday anxiety.

That difference is this: with intuitive guidance, on an inner level, you will *feel* it is right and *know* that if you follow through with action, as hard as it may be, you will be better off. With everyday anxiety, there is no inner safety net giving you the feeling that it will be okay, and so anxiety rises.

Staying in the familiar story of stress, worry or depression can feel easier than having to change. Unfortunately, those feelings will not resolve on their own; they will remain until you decide to act or think differently. Your intuition knows what is best for you in both the short and long term.

If you want to explore your inner wisdom, find a quiet spot and ask yourself what you would like to know, for example, 'what do my feelings need in order to feel calmer?' Then take a few deep, slow breaths in and out, and relax. You may find it easier to close your eyes, or have a pen and paper handy, or focus on a specific thing in front of you.

Be patient, allowing your instincts to present themselves, observing what comes, placing no expectations on a particular outcome. Take note of those first quick feelings, images and 'thoughts', as they usually hold the answers, not the wandering mind chatter. The answers may feel challenging, but deep down, it will feel right.

You may not receive guidance immediately. Like everything, it takes practice and patience. Try not to give up after just one or two goes. Your instincts are with you for life, so it is a good thing to be aware of them and cultivate them.

Treat your intuition like a muscle: the more you use it, the more it develops.

Recognizing what you intuit and following it through with action builds your trust and confidence with your instincts. This will bring alignment between your integrity, beliefs and values, which promotes good mental health.

23.

Empathetic, Sensitive or Empath?

'Some say I'm too sensitive but the truth is I just feel too much. Every word, every action and every energy goes straight to my heart.'

—UNKNOWN

Being sensitive is when someone is open and in tune — whether they know it or not — to all the energy in their environment including the people in it.

We are all like a radio that is constantly receiving and broadcasting energy. Our radio waves, or vibes, are receiving and emitting information 24/7, from and out into our environment. The information contained within those vibes can be about anything, though emotional information is the easiest to pick up on. As our energy is part of the sea of energy that is everywhere, it can tune in, or pick up, and read these energy signals emitting from other people, just as they can pick up and read ours.

Some people are too tuned in, meaning they are very open and sensitive to feeling others' energy. This can make them feel overwhelmed if the people they are open to are feeling anxious, stressed, depressed or in pain. It is possible for them to walk into a room or a mall and pick up someone else's feelings or pain. This is called being an Empath.

The word empath comes from the word empathy, which is the ability to understand the feelings of someone else. For example, your friend tells you her mum is really sick and she is worried. Empathy is what allows you to know the level of emotional pain your friend is going through, even if you have never experienced this type of worry before. However, if you were an empath, you would take things a little further, by sensing, feeling and living your friend's emotions as if they were part of your own experience.

> **This means someone else's pain can become your pain.**

Empathy towards your friends and environment is a wonderful trait to have, though their experiences are for their growth and meant for them in order to learn from. You do not need to take on their emotions. You can listen and offer advice if asked for, but you should not carry, hold or live it.

Therefore, it is important to check in with yourself, seeing if what you are feeling is appropriate for your current circumstances. Is it possible you picked up on someone else's feelings, or are these your own?

Think back to when you first noticed the unusual feelings of sadness, anxiety, depression or whatever the negative feeling is and what was happening at that time. For instance, did it start after you caught up with a friend who was feeling really sad, and you've felt sad since?

Sometimes, just the recognition you may be feeling someone else's anguish or pain is enough to make it disappear as you realise it is not yours to feel or live through.

It is possible to protect yourself against the energy of someone else's pain or anguish from becoming yours. Here are a couple of tips:

When going somewhere that makes you feel uneasy, in your mind, create a visual barrier that completely surrounds you. Imagine that barrier can repel negativity, keeping you safe and protected. It is an energy barrier of intention — the intention of protection.

You could say an affirmation like one the below. Use the words you gel with. You will have better success if the images and words you choose resonate for you.

'The Universe is my shield, guarding me against all negativity.'

'I am safe and protected at all times.'

If you feel you have picked up someone else's anguish, tell yourself the following: *'This is not my worry (or guilt or sadness, whatever the case may be). I no longer need to carry or feel this. It is to be removed from me immediately.'*

You are talking to your energetic aspect that tuned in and picked it up and to your subconscious mind that took it on board and ran with it. You're now telling your energy and subconscious to release and get rid of it. You may need to say it a couple of times, and be quite firm when saying it. Or simply say, *'I release all negative energy from my being.'*

You could follow this by visualizing it being removed from you. For instance, you could see it as a blanket falling off you, or a feather duster flicking away any negative influences.

Saying the words and visualizing it leaving you creates a strong energy of intention for the feelings to be removed.

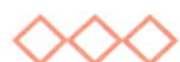

Use your words and images of protection daily until you just naturally feel it is always with you. Use them any time throughout the day, including upon waking and sleeping. Like other practices, it does not stop bad things from happening, though it can reduce the energy of anxiety, depression or pain from someone else becoming yours.

Marie's story

I am nineteen years old. All my life I have felt sensitive to my environment. When I was little, I not only felt it, but my family reinforced it by telling me I was such a 'sensitive little thing'. When I went to school, I felt completely overwhelmed, like I was being bombarded with all sorts of feelings. I didn't really understand it and I didn't like the way it made me feel, so I started imagining I had really tall, strong angels around me who were protecting me so I wouldn't feel that way.

That helped me cope better but it didn't make it easy to make friends, so my school life was quite lonely and anxious. I could easily feel when someone was being genuine or fake, so the other kids did not understand when I didn't want to be around the fake kid, judging me like I wasn't being nice. With so many kids at school and all their emotions, I often found it hard to separate what I was feeling from what I felt from the people around me too.

This stemmed into my work life, but I've now learned more about protecting myself energetically as much as physically. I practise white light surrounding me as well as my angels. I do things to manage my anxiety like exercise, cooking and listening to music, and I definitely check in to see if what I'm feeling is actually mine or real for me.

I still feel other people's emotions, though it doesn't stop me getting out now or making friends as I am much better at protecting myself and recognizing and managing all my senses. Once I realize an emotion is not mine to feel, this starts the process of letting it go. Also, now I'm out of school, I get to pick the environments I want to be in, for example, I have fun supportive friends and where I work has really good vibes with mostly lovely people.

I also say this mantra: 'I have a light inside me that protects me always, keeping me strong and safe.' This has really helped. It took a while to feel those words, but I do now.

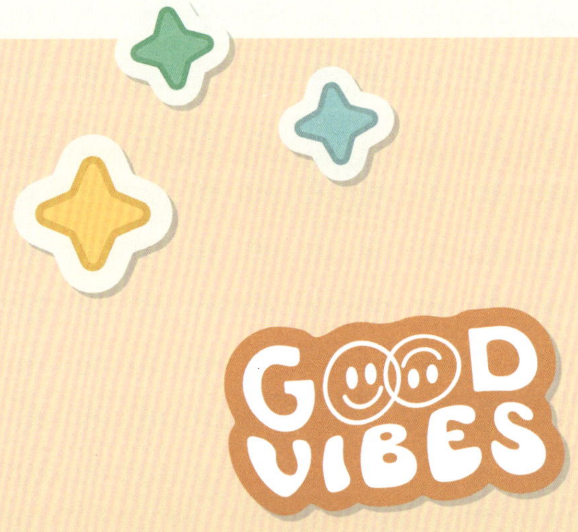

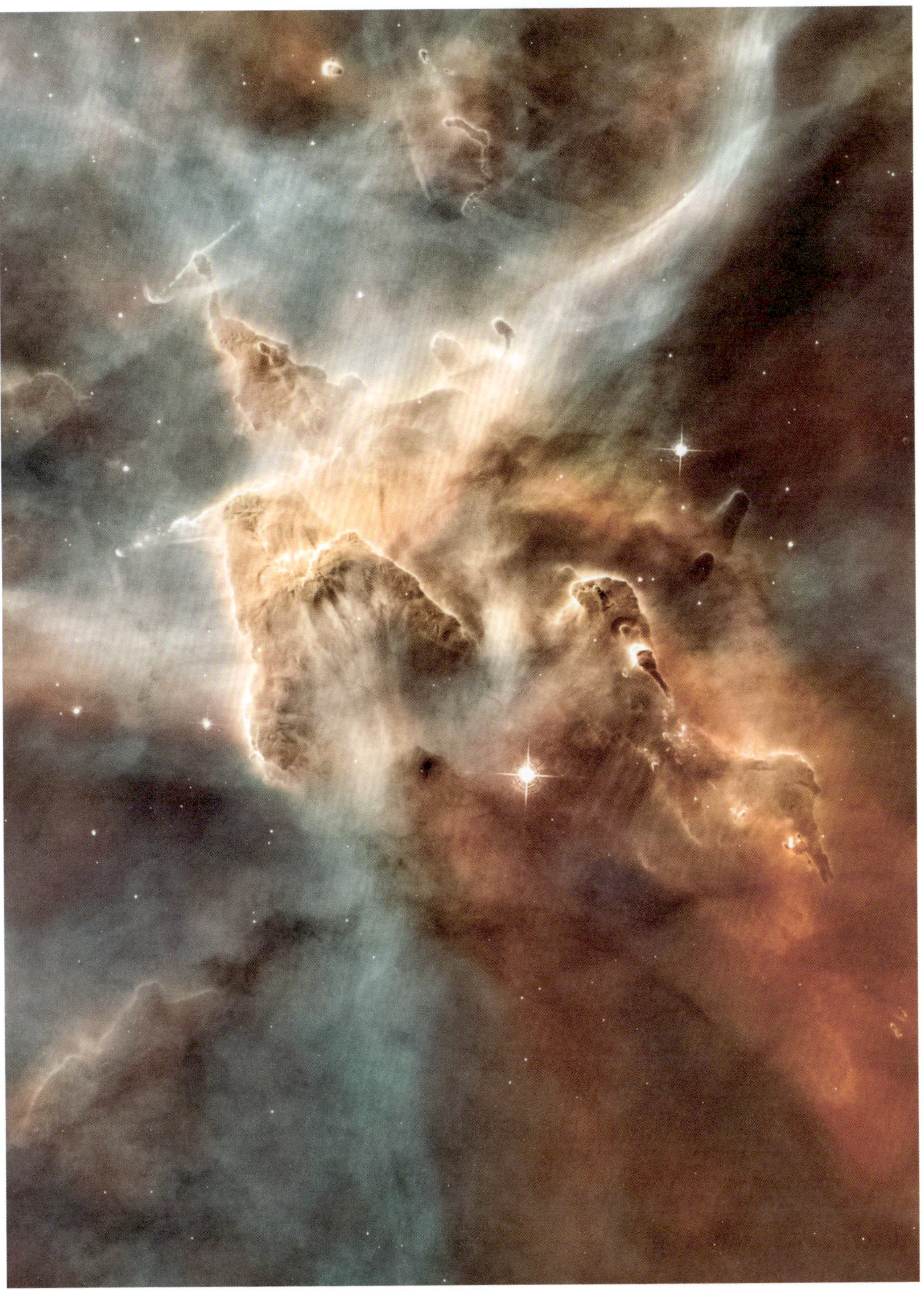

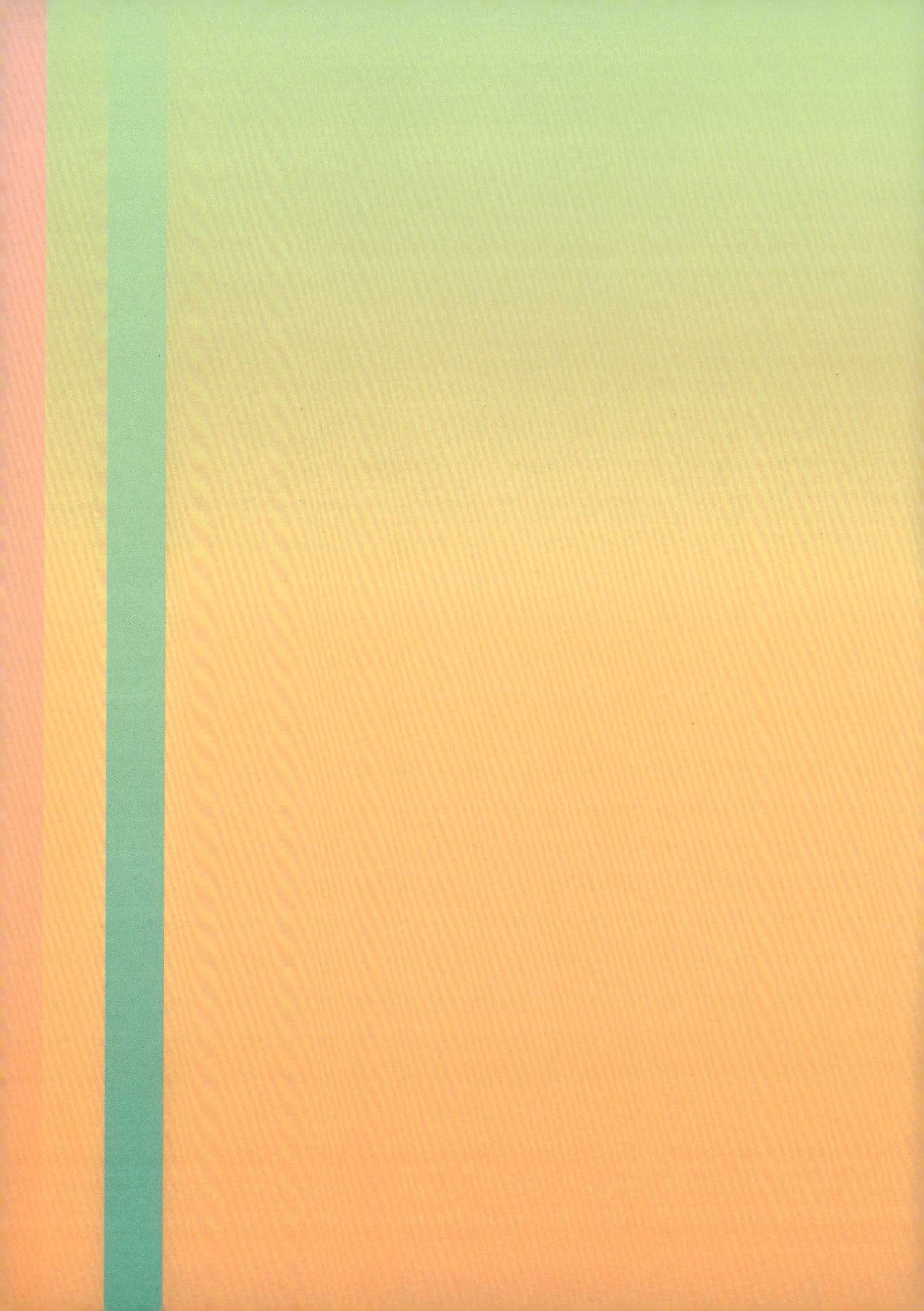

The DIETARY Toolkit

24.

The Gut/Brain/ Immune Connection

'Let food be thy medicine and medicine be thy food.'

—HIPPOCRATES

The saying 'you are what you eat' is literally true. The nutrients in our food get broken down and absorbed into our body to provide it with the fuel it needs to function properly. Depending on what we consume, this can lead us to be physically, mentally and emotionally healthy, or less so.

This is because most of our immune cells are found in our gut, along with hundreds of millions of neurotransmitters (nervous system cells) that help stabilize our mood and make us feel good.

They can actively and independently think and feel just like our brain can; hence, our gut is often referred to as our second brain.

Basically, it means the function of these three body systems can affect each other due to their location, creating the gut/brain/immune connection.

This makes our food choices very important, as they will not only affect our gut function, but also our immune and mood as well and vice versa. Essentially, healthy foods and beverages lead to good gut, immune and mental function, and unhealthy foods and beverages lead to poor gut, immune and mental function.

It also means that improving one will improve the others too. Good mental health helps good gut function; good gut function helps our mood.

We have looked at tools to directly help our beliefs, thoughts and energy, now let's look at how our diet also helps our mental health, as healthy foods may be different for everyone.

25.

Food Sensitivities

Foods that leave us feeling tired, bloated or with a sore stomach may mean our body is sensitive to them. It is easy to determine if we have a food allergy through blood tests or a skin prick test. However, a food sensitivity is more difficult as it is often a smaller reaction and can take up to 24 hours before any symptoms present. Though, if it is a food we consume regularly, it's possible to have persistent symptoms.

Symptoms can occur if the immune cells located in our gut perceive a particular food as not right for us, like it's a foreign body, and, if so, it will generate an immune response against it. That usually involves the release of chemicals such as histamine and the production of inflammation. Inflammation in the gut hinders the breakdown of our food into useful chemicals that are beneficial for good mental health.

This frequently happens when we are stressed, anxious, sad or overwhelmed and so on, as these feelings put us into our fight or flight mode, which, in turn, dials down our gut function as it is not needed when the body is dealing with the stress. Since most of our immune cells are located in the gut, their function is also dialled down, making it difficult for them to determine which foods are okay for us or not.

Food sensitivity symptoms include tiredness, brain fog, poor concentration, loose bowels, constipation, bloating, stomach aches, eczema, hay fever, acne and low mood. They may also exacerbate any spectrum disorders such as ADHD.

If you would like to know what foods you may be sensitive to, an elimination diet can help. It involves eliminating one food group for three weeks then slowly re-introducing it to see how it makes you feel: tired, brain fog, dizziness, skin breakouts, tummy upset, headaches and so on — it could be anything. All symptoms are our body's way of saying, for whatever reason, 'I do not like that food.'

I highly recommend talking with a qualified naturopath to design a good elimination programme as they can design it specifically for you and your needs. Dietary requirements vary for each person depending on their lifestyle or medical history, for example those with diabetes.

Some naturopaths can do a food sensitivity test through hair analysis, which may be easier and a lot quicker! A very small sample of hair is cut and sent off for examination for food and environmental sensitivities, using an EAV machine.

However, if you would like to try elimination, here are the things to consider.

The first thing to do is to plan. Before starting, check each food group and know exactly what foods you will be avoiding and what foods you may need to increase or add to ensure you maintain enough protein, carbohydrates and good fats, along with high nutrient dense foods (lots of vegetables). You may need to look at new menus/recipes.

It is also important to consider whether it is a good time to start an elimination diet. Are there any upcoming events or travel plans that may interfere with the diet? Do you have the determination and energy to carry it out, as it will take some time to complete? Do you feel comfortable with temporary food limitations? Do you have support from family and friends?

If you feel you are ready to start, your naturopath will most likely advise you to do the following steps. Continue with your normal diet as much as possible while completely stopping one of the food groups below for three weeks, then afterwards, slowly re-introduce it over the next three days. As you do, take note of how you feel. If you feel okay, continue eating it and move to the next food group and so on until all the food groups have had a three-week elimination period followed by a three-day re-introduction period.

If at any stage when re-introducing a food, you feel unwell or have a reaction to it, even a small one, stop eating it, as this may indicate a food sensitivity. Once you feel better, start eliminating the next food group, as it's possible to have more than one food sensitivity. If you accidently eat a food you are avoiding, then you will need to start the three-week process again.

When you have finished the whole process, try reintroducing the foods you noticed you had a reaction to occasionally to see how you feel. It may be that you can tolerate a little without symptoms. You can choose the order of which foods you wish to eliminate:

Dairy: Includes milk, cheese, cream, ice-cream, sour cream, cream cheese, yoghurt, whey protein powder, milk solids and foods containing dairy such as milo and chocolate.

Sugars: White and brown sugars, jams, honey, caster sugar, icing sugar, rice syrup, maple syrup and golden syrup. Foods such as biscuits, cakes, lollies, some cereals, fizzy drinks and fruit juices.

Gluten: Includes flour, cereals, breads, pasta, biscuits, crackers, cakes and any other items in the cupboard with flour or gluten in them. Note, you may use gluten free options to replace them with.

Eggs.

Soy products: Milk, cheese, ice-cream, yoghurt, tofu, miso soup.

Caffeine: Coffee, black and green tea, fizzy and energy drinks and chocolate. Also check supplements taken for weight loss or to help gym workouts.

Meats: Chicken, pork, lamb, beef (steak and mince), bacon. Stop the meats you regularly consume one at a time followed by a reintroduction period — do this for each meat type. Ensure you eat other sources of protein throughout your day while not eating meats. For example, eggs, nuts, seeds, chick peas, quinoa, tofu, beans and oats.

Fish: Stop the seafood you regularly consume, one at a time for three weeks, followed by a three-day re-introduction period.

Fruits: Stop each fruit you consume regularly one at a time followed by the three-day re-introduction period.

Vegetables: Stop each vegetable you consume regularly one at a time followed by the three-day reintroduction period.

Other: Stop any other foods you regularly consume, such as nuts or seeds or anything not mentioned above, for the three-week elimination period followed by the three-day re-introduction.

If you want to feel good, with lots of energy, you have to consider the best fuel for your body in order to run it. You would not put petrol into a diesel car and expect it to work fine.

26.

Beneficial Nutrients

'To keep the body in good health is a duty ... otherwise we shall not be able to keep our mind strong and clear.'

—BUDDHA

Our food should provide us with all the nutrients we need for our physical, mental and emotional wellbeing.

As a general rule, this involves eating a wide range of colourful vegetables: two servings of fruit a day (one serve is the size of one of your cupped hands); proteins from meat, chicken, eggs, nuts, seeds, chick peas, beans, quinoa, oats or tofu; carbohydrates such as starchy vegetables like potato and pumpkin or small amount of brown rice or pasta; healthy fats such as avocado, nuts and seeds; and plenty of water.

The *occasional* treat can also be added into the mix, like something sweet or a takeaway. It can be difficult to avoid the many fast-food options, as they advertise prolifically, are often cheap and they add a lot of sugar substances and salt to tantalize the taste buds, making them rather addictive to our palette — see Food Additives on page 111. If you like a slice of pizza or a hamburger, try making them at home from fresh products.

Consuming enough vitamins and minerals from our foods has become increasingly more difficult for several reasons. Over-cultivation of crops on the same soil depletes the nutrients from it and therefore less get into our food; pesticides strip minerals from the soil; and fruits and vegetables are often picked before they fully ripen in order to get them to the consumer.

Supplementation can be a good way to ensure we get the right nutrients, especially if we are deficient in one or more. The best way to check nutrient deficiencies is a blood test, though not all can be tested and may cost money to do so. The idea is to use the supplement(s) until your bloods show you are decently within the normal ranges *and* your symptoms have improved. After that, use food to maintain a balanced nutrient rich diet.

A qualified naturopath or your doctor can organize blood tests for you and can advise on any necessary supplementation once they have the results.

Nutrients that are important for good mental health are:

Tryptophan: This nutrient is an essential amino acid and our body needs it to make the chemicals, serotonin, our happy hormone, and melatonin, our sleep hormone. Unfortunately, our body cannot make it. Therefore, this essential nutrient must come from our diet. Symptoms of low tryptophan in our body include anxiety, depression, irritability, increased pain sensitivity, poor concentration, sleep disturbances, insomnia and acoustic startle. Foods high in tryptophan are chicken, eggs, pumpkin and sesame seeds, walnuts, cashews, tofu and fish.

Vitamin C: This vitamin keeps our immune system working properly during times of stress. It helps iron absorption, which reduces fatigue and it is one of the main nutrients needed for good adrenal gland function. Our adrenals release a variety of hormones that run our body including regulating our fight or flight response. Foods high in Vitamin C include oranges and orange juice, lemons, grapefruit, peppers, strawberries, broccoli, Brussels sprouts and blackcurrants.

Vitamin B complex: All B vitamins are necessary for our health and the proper functioning of the nervous system, especially when stressed, and they are essential for maintaining energy levels. Chicken, eggs and whole grains are rich in a variety of B vitamins.

Pernicious anaemia is a deficiency in the production of red blood cells due to a lack of vitamin B12, which may cause tiredness or more seriously, if left undiagnosed, may result in permanent neurological damage. Vitamin B12 is chiefly found in meat and fish. Some cereals, breads and dairy products may have it added to their ingredients (it will say fortified with B12 on the packaging). If you are vegetarian or vegan, you should check your B12 levels with regular blood tests.

Vitamin D: Research indicates Vitamin D has an important role in guarding against depression and regulating mood. Ninety per cent of our vitamin D comes from exposure to sunlight on our bare (un-sunblocked) skin. Very little comes from our food.

It works like this: the sunlight on our skin generates the production of 'inactive' vitamin D, which then travels through our blood to our kidneys and liver, where enzymes convert it to its 'active' form. Therefore, try to get fifteen to 20 minutes of sun exposure (without sunblock) on your arms, face or legs every day when the sun will not burn you.

Note, there is a small percentage of the population who cannot convert the sun's rays on their skin; therefore, a supplement would be needed. Again, get a blood test first to check and, if low, use a sublingual Vitamin D supplement such as a spray or dissolvable tablet that goes under your tongue, as it will absorb straight into the blood vessels located there, rather than through the gut and then absorbed into the blood.

Magnesium: This plays a key role in determining how much vitamin D our body can make as it appears to be needed to activate vitamin D. It also relaxes the nervous system and muscles. If supplementing with both magnesium and vitamin D, take them at the same time; if just taking magnesium, this is better taken at night after a meal for better absorption and to help make the sleep hormone, melatonin. Symptoms of a magnesium deficiency include insomnia, jitteriness, anxiety, heart palpitations, headaches, constipation and sore/cramping muscles. Green vegetables, almonds, kelp, wheat germ, sesame seeds and fish are rich in this mineral.

Iron: Adequate iron is needed to form our blood. Our blood carries oxygen to every cell and organ in our body. Ferritin is our stored iron. Anaemia, meaning low iron levels, puts a physical stress on the body, resulting in symptoms such as fatigue, irritability, brain fog and poor concentration. Often those diagnosed with ADHD are low in iron. It is different from pernicious anaemia, which is indicated with low B12 levels, though initially the symptoms may appear similar.

Good sources of iron include red meats such as beef, lamb and pork, dark green leafy vegetables such as spinach, seafood, beans, peas, dried fruits such as raisins and apricots, as well as iron-fortified (meaning added) foods like cereal, bread and pasta.

If supplementing with iron, choose one that also contains vitamin C as it helps the iron to be absorbed properly through the digestive system. If it is not absorbed properly, this can lead to constipation. Do not take your iron supplement while drinking a cup of tea, as the tannins found in regular tea hinder the absorption.

Note, more and more people are suffering from low iron for a variety of reasons. Do not assume that if you are male or eat lots of red meat your iron levels will be fine. If you feel consistently tired or find it difficult to concentrate at school, it's good to get it checked.

27.

Food Additives

'The foods you eat can either be the safest and most powerful of medicine, or the slowest form of poison.'

—ANN WIGMORE

The production of food additives is a billion-dollar industry, in particular creating artificial sweeteners, flavours and colours (dyes). These all contain substances that may be considered neurotoxic, meaning they are harmful to our brain function.

For an example of how additives can affect us, think about what happens when a child drinks a bottle of flavoured, fluorescent-coloured fizzy drink along with a bag of colourful lollies. The artificial sugars, flavours and dyes promptly stimulate the gut nerve cells, which affect the child's behaviour, putting them into supernova drive!

We all know that rainbow-coloured fruits and vegetables are good for us. This may be why bright artificial colours are added to unhealthy foods and drinks to make us think the food is actually good for us. For example, custard is a diluted yellow colour bordering on beige, yet most custard squares from a bakery are bright yellow due to the added yellow dye to make them look more appealing.

Artificial sweeteners and flavours like aspartame, saccharine and MSG are added to entice our taste buds so we cannot help but bite into the unhealthy refined foods and beverages. This industry knows our taste buds from our hunter-gather days are still hardwired to crave those sweet foods that were in short supply back then. Therefore, it might not be a good idea to trust the messages our taste buds are communicating to us!

Despite being widely used, 80 per cent of all adverse reactions to food additives reported to the US Food and Drugs Administration (FDA) concerned aspartame. These reactions have included headaches, migraines, dizziness, seizures, nausea, muscle spasm, weight gain, rashes, depression, fatigue, irritability, and tachycardia, vision problems, breathing difficulties, anxiety attacks, vertigo, tinnitus, memory loss and joint pain.

Many people consume energy drinks as the labelling is enticing, all their friends drink them or they love the taste due to the intense sweetness (from the artificial sweeteners) and like the energy or wired feeling (from the artificial colours) it gives them. As the dyes and artificial sweeteners are neurotoxins, they can disrupt our normal nervous system function, leading to increased symptoms of irritability, anxiety and depression.

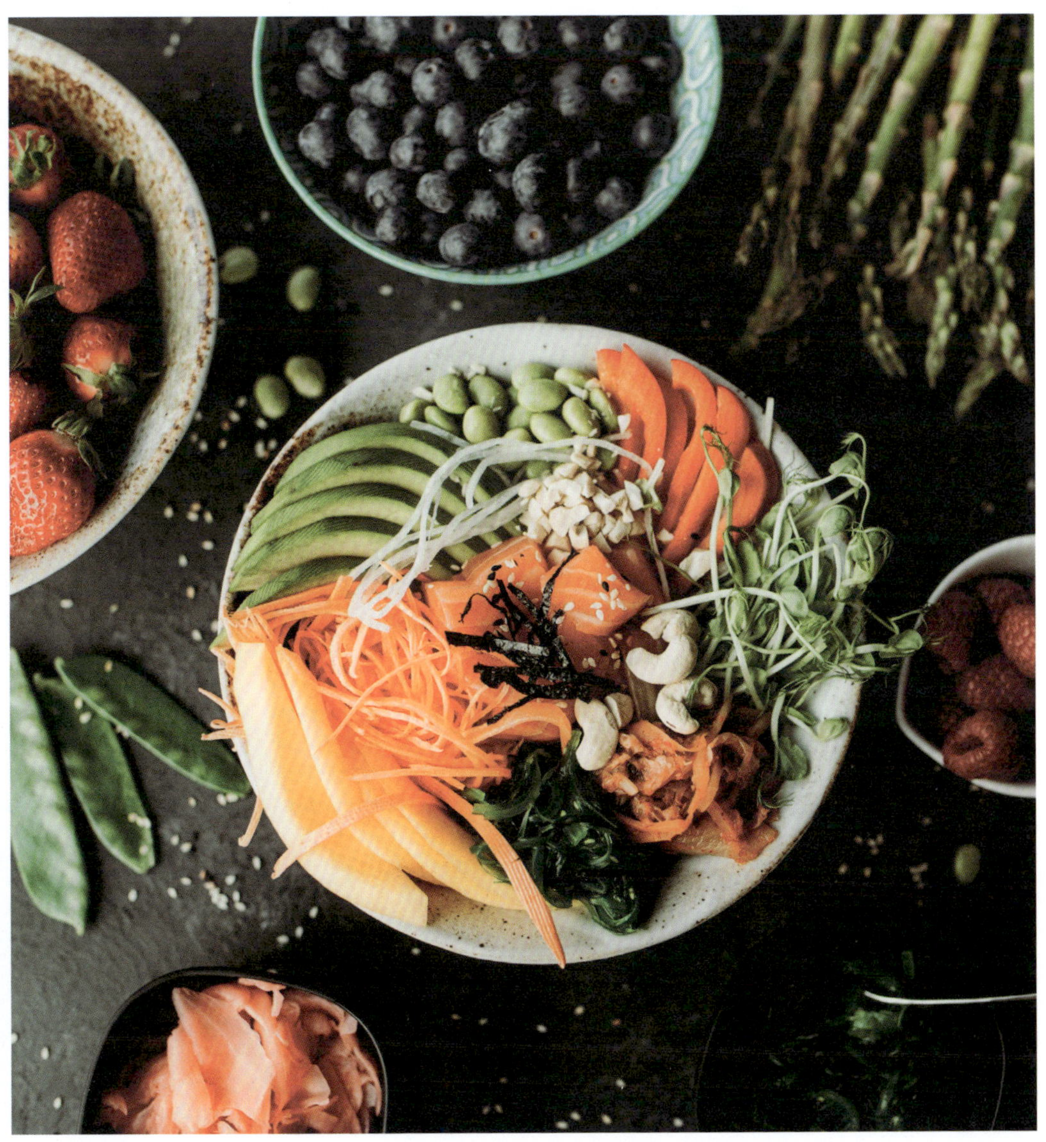

Maddy's story

I started drinking energy drinks every day when I was studying for my end-of-year exams and continued drinking them. The next year, I noticed my anxiety was getting worse and I also started getting migraines and had to take a day or two off school every few weeks, which made me worry more. My mum took me to a naturopath, who suggested a few changes in my diet and recommended magnesium and herbs to ease my anxiety and migraines. But before we did any of that, she recommended I stop the energy drinks to see if that fixed the problem. She told me the aspartame found in energy drinks can cause headaches and migraines in some sensitive people, as well as worsen anxiety and insomnia.

As I did not want the herbs, I agreed to stop the energy drinks. My anxiety did not fully go, but it didn't feel as out of control as it had been, and the migraines completely stopped.

I now look for aspartame in everything I buy as I do not want to feel like that again and I'm a lot more aware of listening to my body about what foods it does and doesn't like.

The nasty additives

There are many types of food additives and a long list of harmful ones. These are a few of the particularly harmful ones found in everyday foods. Each has an international number attributed to it and in Europe they put an 'E' in front of the number. It is the number you need to look for.

Artificial colours: to add colour

E102 Tartrazine
E104 Quinoline yellow
E107 Yellow 2G
E110 Sunset yellow
E122 Azorubine, carmoisine
E123 Amaranth, purplish red
E124 Ponceau, brilliant scarlet
E127 Erythrosine, cherry pink/red
E128 Red 2G
E129 Allure red
E132 Indigotine, indigo carmine
E133 Brilliant blue
E142 Green S, food green, acid brilliant green
E151 Brilliant black
E155 Brown, chocolate brown

Oxidizing agent: used to raise foods like breads

E924 Potassium bromate

Preservatives: keep foods from changing colour, changing the flavour or going off (rancid)

E210, E211, E212, E213 Benzoates
E220, E221, E222, E223, Sulphites
E250, E251 Nitrates
E320 Butylated hydroxyanisole (BHA)
E321 Butylated hydroxytoluene (BHT)

Artificial sweeteners

E951 Aspartame
E954 Saccharin
E950 Acesulfame-K

28.

Herbs for Health

The use of herbs for our health and in our cooking for flavour has been around since hunter-gatherer times. Herbal medicines, along with healthy eating and lifestyle factors, have increasingly been shown to be valid treatment options for many health concerns. Herbal medicine is one of the oldest forms of medicine and is still one of the main treatments for most of the population in the world, especially in non-western countries.

Herbs are considered to be safe, effective and evidence-based natural remedies. Some herbs have contraindications or cautions as they may interact with various medications or with some health concerns. They have little or no side effects, though, like everything, there is no rule that one size fits all.

As a clinical naturopath, medical herbalist and as a supervisor at the largest Natural Medicinal Colleges in New Zealand, the proof is in the pudding. Meaning, I have seen over and over, with hundreds and hundreds of clients, how effective herbal and nutritional medicine is in helping people reduce their mental, emotional and physical health concerns.

If you wish to look at herbs to improve mental health and reduce stress levels, I highly recommend you see a qualified naturopath who is also a qualified medical herbalist. If you are on any medications, they will also ensure any recommended herbs are not contraindicated with them.

Over-the-counter herbs that are beneficial to support our mental health can be found in herbal teas and supplements. Not all supplements are created equally and some find herbal tea not strong enough to make a significant difference, though some find them soothing and calming, which helps aid their digestion and sleep. If you would like to try a herbal tea, some herbs to look for are listed below.

Note, if you have any concerns regarding a herbal supplement, please discuss this with your doctor or a qualified naturopath/ medical herbalist.

Anxiolytic (reduces anxiety)

Passionflower, Bacopa, Californian Poppy, Valerian

Stress relief

Ashwaganda (also known as Withania), Rhodiola, Oats, Chamomile, some Ginsengs

Anti-depressant

Rhodiola, Saffron or St John's Wort (cannot have if taking anti-depressant medication)

Calming and supporting the nervous and digestive systems

Chamomile, Oats, Lemon Balm, Peppermint, Ginger (take with caution if using blood thinner medications)

Adrenal support

Rehmannia or Liquorice (cannot have if on blood pressure medication)

Improve mental cognitive function

Bacopa, Lion's Mane

Improve sleep

Californian Poppy, Spiny Jujube (also known as Zizyphus), Valerian, Oats, Lemon Balm, Skullcap

The LIFESTYLE Toolkit

29.

Sleep

No matter how old we are, sleep is vital! We all know that poor quality and inadequate sleep leaves us tired and cranky.

Quality sleep has a profound effect on our physical, mental, emotional and social development, as it:

- repairs physical damage
- benefits our mental capacity, as it promotes memory, attention and analytical thinking
- improves our emotional status by regulating hormones
- aids our social status, as poor sleep leads to irritability and exaggerated emotional reactions.

It has been shown that teenagers typically need between eight to ten hours of sleep every night and seven and a half to eight hours per night once past the teenage years. If it is consistently less than that, it is deemed sleep deprivation.

Sleep deprivation can have dramatic detrimental effects on our mental wellbeing and academic/performance pressures. It may negatively affect emotional development, which, thereby, increases the risks for interpersonal conflict and the more serious mental health issues of anxiety, depression, insomnia and bipolar disorder, which have all been linked to poor sleep.

Good sleep hygiene cannot be underestimated. If you are not consistently getting enough quality sleep every night, here are some tips you may find helpful:

For 30 to 60 minutes before bed, stop looking at screens: laptops, computers and phones. The blue light from these devices may trigger a physical response in our brain that maintains wakefulness.

Create a cooler, quiet, dark room to sleep in. Ensure the temperature is right for you and try an eye mask and/or ear plugs if it is not quite dark or quiet enough. Sometimes even when it is, they can still be beneficial as it can be a 'cue' to your brain to be quiet.

For some, having soft white noise (calming consistent noise) like a fan blowing is better than silence.

A heavy blanket can be soothing, as it gives a safe, comfy feeling. There are specifically designed blankets to improve sleep and anxiety. Search for 'calming blanket' or 'therapy blanket'.

Do not drink any caffeinated drinks after 3 p.m. as they are a stimulant that promotes wakefulness. These include energy drinks, cola (and a lot of other fizzy drinks), coffee, black or green tea (other herbal teas are okay). There are various herbal teas you could have before bed to help drift into sleep, like chamomile, lavender, lemon balm, valerian and oats, or something with a combination of these.

A sleep meditation can help quieten the mind, allowing you to drift off to sleep. There are many meditation apps available, like Insight Timer and the one on my website: www.nicolalincoln.co.nz

Lavender helps promote sleep. Have a warm bath with lavender essential oil, or spray it on a tissue and place on your pillow — do not put an essential oil directly onto your skin, as it needs to be put in a carrier oil or diluted in water.

To help increase your natural melatonin, try a magnesium supplement, one hour before bed. It needs to be a minimum of 400 mg of elemental (or equivalent) magnesium.

Eye exercises help the eyes close and relax as well as distract the mind. With eyes open or closed, flick your eyes up ten times, then down ten times, to the right ten times and then to your left ten times. Repeat until you want to stop.

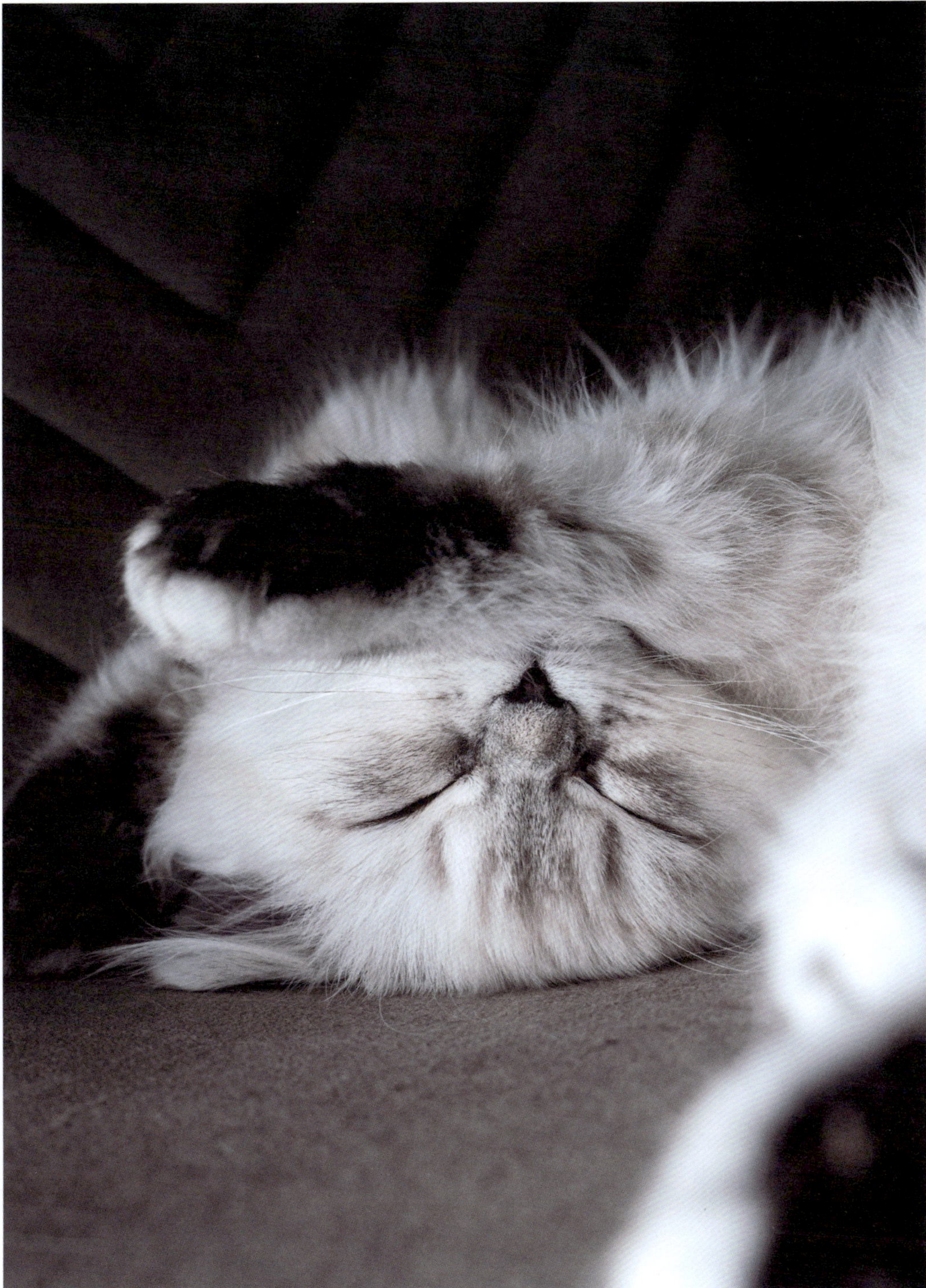

30.

Exercise

We all know exercise is good for our health and it can boost our confidence if feeling and looking fit and healthy is important to us. When we exercise, our body creates endorphins, which interact with the receptors in our brain that reduce our perception of pain. They can also trigger a positive feeling in our body by energising our spirits, which is why we often feel good or 'high' after exercise, as our energy has increased — not just relief that it's finished!

It improves mental health by reducing stress, anxiety and depression, while lifting our mood and energy, improving self-esteem and cognitive function, and supporting better sleep hygiene. It encourages various changes within our brain such as promoting neural growth and feelings of calmness and wellbeing.

The even better news is, you do not have to be a fitness junkie or fanatic to reap the benefits. No matter what your fitness level is, you can use exercise as a great tool to cope with various mental health concerns, and improve your energy and outlook on life. Pick something you enjoy doing, as you are more likely to stick with it.

It is recommended that teens do 60 minutes of moderate, aerobic exercise every day — which means anything that gets the heart pumping a little, or a lot. If you're not big on team sports or the gym, pick something else you enjoy, like putting music on in your room and dancing around for a while.

There are many studies that show exercise works as effectively as anti-anxiety and anti-depression medication, but without the nasty side effects. It is a natural and effective way to help with all mental health issues.

Get moving! You don't have to join a gym, though you can if that interests you. If not, there are lots of other forms of exercise you can do at home if shyness or perhaps cost are factors.

Use your own body weight as resistance training rather than weights/equipment. Do some sit ups, squats, push ups, lunges, tricep dips, skipping rope, and star jumps. Before you start, watch some good YouTube clips to show you how to do them safely. If you're shaking your head at this, then pick something you enjoy doing so it does not feel like exercise, but feels fun. This could include roller blading, ice skating (or any type of skating), shooting hoops, power walking the dog or dancing. You always feel better after you finish exercising! Puffed maybe, but good!

31.

Social Media is Not Your Therapist

'Engage, enlighten, encourage and especially ... Just be yourself. Social media is a community effort, everyone is an asset.'

—SUSAN COOPER

Social media was designed as a way of exchanging information, ideas and photos through a virtual community, in particular between friends and family who live far away from each other. It helps them to still feel connected and part of each other's lives. Now we exchange those same things with someone who is sitting right next to us. It has become a common way to communicate with one another, whether far away or nearby.

Since the internet started, we have had access to all sorts of heath information. In the late 1990s Google, nicknamed, 'Doctor Google', allowed people to type in their symptoms to see if they were bad enough to go and visit the doctor. Then social media exploded on a variety of platforms with billions of clips and posts of people expressing their symptoms and labelling them as a particular health concern like anxiety, borderline personality disorder (BPD), depression, dyslexia and so on. On TikTok alone *#anxiety* currently has 22 billion views.

This has certainly helped to remove the stigma around mental health anguish. After hearing other people's stories, we are now more open and okay with seeking help. Access to this free information can reduce the risk of feeling embarrassed, or from being rejected when speaking to a teacher or parent. It can also help us feel like we're not alone, especially in those dark times. This alone can save lives.

However, if that content is focused on someone else's problems, without sharing what tools or strategies helped them, it may leave the viewer feeling even more lost or that everything is hopeless.

It is important to note, most of this content is not created by a mental health expert, but every day, ordinary people. And to add to that, it is built on algorithms. When you type in what you are interested in like, 'how do I cope with depression?', you will be bombarded with an endless stream of similar content thereafter. This can amplify emotions, making everything seem larger and scarier than it actually is if it's always in your face.

For some, it has become common to view a *diagnostic* mental health concern as part of their identity, rather than viewing it as a period in their lives. It's talked about in such a casual manner like, 'Yeah I've had anxiety all my life.' This is particularly concerning if they are the creator of their own diagnosis.

When we self-diagnose, we may take on potentially misleading or limited information that draws an incomplete picture, leaving us with incorrect conclusions and perceptions regarding our wellbeing. This may lead to labelling ourselves with a mental health condition when, in fact, we are just experiencing normal, healthy emotions associated with the various challenges in our lives.

If your thoughts and feelings are stopping you from having a contented, happy life, then I encourage you to reach out to someone you know, a trusted family member, friend, teacher or school counsellor. The aim is for them to provide you with a different perspective on your situation, thoughts or feelings, rather than through social media, which knows nothing of your personal background or history.

Social media has also created a perception that some people live perfect lives, according to their posts. The reality is, no one has a perfect life. Yet we still constantly compare ourselves to others regardless of if it's real or not. This can promote feelings of jealousy or inadequacy that may trigger intrusive, depressive or anxious thoughts.

Bear this in mind when you next look at your various news or social media platforms, especially if you are feeling low. Maybe take a break from scrolling through that day to reduce these feelings. It will still be there tomorrow — and tomorrow, you may be able to view it through a different filter if you are feeling happier and more confident within yourself.

No doubt, social media plays a big role in shaping our lives. Like everything, it can be empowering and uplifting or limiting and damaging. But *you get to choose* how and when you wish to engage with it.

Noah's story

There are two different events to mark the 'beginning' of my anxiety. First, I'd say at the age of thirteen it was triggered by an event where I woke up in the night after having some weird dream where there were flashing lights and random shapes. Not sure exactly what spooked me about it so much, but from then on, I started having sleeping problems and I would get upset when bedtime came around. I didn't exactly see it as anxiety at the time, but now I look back on it, it definitely was.

I went to see someone about it and I guess it sort of helped, but personally I am not a huge fan of therapists and such. I still sometimes have sleeping problems today; it comes and goes sporadically.

Then at the age of fifteen, one day after being out with my mum at the movies, my body basically broke down and started aching everywhere. I constantly felt in pain, even though there was nothing physically wrong with me. This kept happening in different ways for over a year before I started realizing it was probably the anxiety causing this. That did make it better, because I think I had subconsciously convinced myself it was something worse, which was in fact actually making the pains more frequent. I would constantly search on the internet for answers to my pains, which told me very disturbing things. At times I felt helpless and thought I had to live with the pains forever.

I definitely felt worse if something relating to the things I feared or to the triggering event came up in conversation. Along with health worries, I also fear different aspects of the future such as climate change (nuclear war was another big one a few years ago) so I would, and I still do try to, avoid politics and current world affairs. Also, this is quite specific, but Twitter has an explore page where it has a list of current affairs in the world, so I became 'addicted' to checking what was going on in the world. Although I wanted to avoid it, sometimes it became hard to do so. I have had OCD as well from a young age, so it definitely didn't help with my negative thoughts.

Now I am nineteen years old, I am at university, I have a solid support system, close friends ... Yet do I feel entirely okay? No, definitely not. I'm still fearful of my future, but I can definitely say I am better off than where I was a few years ago. I am on medication but I don't really meditate or do any of those rituals to help it. If I am anxious, sometimes I will watch a show that makes me happy in an attempt to lighten my mood and I have become more selective of when and what I view on my media platforms.

32.

For Safety's Sake

There are many things in our lives and in the world that can make us feel unsafe. Conflict between countries, random acts of terror at our schools, malls, concerts to name a few, through to feeling unsafe at school from bullying behaviours and unrest at home with families struggling to make ends meet, or with divorce or neglect.

In most cases these things are outside our control. What we can control is how we wish to react to them to manage our feelings, or we can speak up, advocating for change.

Neither of these are easy to do. We will always automatically react in the same fashion as we always have. It means we have to consciously stop and review the situation before we react. This is when those deep, long breaths can help! (See Mindfulness on page 64.) Speaking up when we are fearful of the consequence, or lack confidence to do so, is also challenging.

Feeling unsafe or scared for a moment or for extended periods of time is stressful and can cause or worsen any mental health concern. Here is a range of topics and tips to help you feel safe.

Bullying

Bullying behaviours occur because often bullies themselves have been, or are being, bullied. You do not generally see happy people going around hurting others. Hurt people are the ones who go on to hurt other people. This does not excuse their behaviour, yet, to change, they need better role models in their lives, teaching them love, compassion and kindness. If they are overly mean, often they have misplaced anger and frustration as they have not learned healthy coping behaviours.

Some bullies are either envious, jealous of what you have and deal with this by putting you down. Or they project their own insecurities onto you, making fun of you for the very thing they are insecure about.

If someone is mean to you, remember, this is not about you.

> **Start seeing how they treat you as a reflection of who they truly are and not a measure of your worthiness.**

Then there are those self-absorbed bullies, who are so focused on themselves, they have no awareness of how their words or actions may affect others.

'Ignore the people who talk behind your back. That's where they belong; behind you.'

—DR JULIE CONNER

If you are being harassed by a bully, here are some tips for you to try:

Bullies tend to target those they think are weak. Try acting as if your self-confidence is strong. Act proud of who you are, walking with your head held high.

Take a positive stance against the person by taking charge of your space and calling out their behaviour. If it is physical bullying, loudly say their name and tell them to stop hurting you, as shouting draws unwanted attention to them. If it is verbal, try to stay calm and not react – bullies often want you to engage as this is like an invitation for them to continue.

When in a group of people, if someone says something mean, degrading or upsetting to you, turn it around by asking them clearly, 'Are you okay?' This sends a message to them and the group, that their behaviour is *not* okay, and it also robs them of the satisfaction of a reaction from you.

Stay with a crowd; try not to get isolated. Follow others into the bathroom, sit with or near others at break times or walk with others to classes and in and out of school.

Talk with a trustworthy adult: parent, teacher, counsellor, coach, even your bus driver if you take the bus to school and that's where the bullying occurs. Bullies want you to believe that talking to an adult makes you a coward. This is to stop you from doing it, as if you do, then they will be held accountable.

Affirmation: *'I am worthy, courageous and strong.'* Say this three times in a row, many times throughout your day for three weeks, or until you feel you no longer need it.

Home life

Home should be a safe space where everyone feels accepted, supported, cared for and loved — no matter what! For some, this is not the case.

Pressures may arise due to various family dynamics from parents separating through to high expectations of performance in academics, sports or the arts, which may adversely affect mental and emotional health.

Society has come to expect instant results and gratification, and this can put additional, sometimes unfair, pressure and expectations on young people. A lot of this pressure comes from well-meaning parents and teachers, but what is the right balance between encouragement and expectation?

If you are feeling upset or unsure at home here are some suggestions for you:

If parents are putting unfair or too much pressure on you to perform well at school, in sport or in the arts, to the point where it is negatively feeding into your mental and emotional wellbeing, it's time to let them know. Parents who do this usually do so as they want the best for you, which is always better than not caring at all. However, if their expectations and judgements are leading you to believe you are not good enough, or make you feel anxious, down or scared, it's important to let them know.

If this is difficult to do, it may help to talk it through with a teacher, school counsellor or another trusted adult who can help you discuss your feelings with your parents.

If parents are arguing or are mean to each other in front of you, let them know it upsets you. Your feelings matter; therefore, by letting them know, they should either act better around you or leave the room.

You do not have to take sides if your parents separate. They may act in a way that makes you feel you have to, but let them know that you should be allowed to be with either parent without the other getting mad, hurt or jealous.

Continue your study, after-school activities, part-time job or seeing friends. When home life is stressful or changing, it can be good to maintain normality in other areas of your life.

Affirmation: *'I am enough and deserve respect and kindness.'* Say this three times in a row, many times throughout your day for three weeks, or until you feel you no longer need it.

Friendships

Feeling like we fit in and belong is a key factor to our mental and emotional health. We thrive when we have like-minded people around us, as this helps us feel worthy, supported and safe. Friendships offer a real connection based on mutual respect, kindness and love. It is not about who we spend the *most* time with, but who we have the *best* time with.

If we believe we do not fit in or have genuine friendships, it may result in feeling withdrawn and disconnected with our environment and the people in it. Feeling withdrawn and disconnected are known risk factors for depression and anxiety, and if left unresolved for too long, potentially, this may lead to unhealthy coping behaviours.

Fitting in and belonging is such a cornerstone of our psyche that we will often form friendships with others who do not support us, who do not align with our integrity or who are simply just not nice people. *It is vital to recognize genuine friendship over disingenuous or harmful ones for your emotional safety.* It is important to let go of friends who make you question yourself or make you unhappy, and try to meet new people who share the same interests as you.

Never worry about losing a friend — a real friend can never be lost, and your best friends will be the people who make your problems their problems, so you do not have to go it alone.

The ideas below have been mentioned throughout the book, though it is worth mentioning them again, as finding your tribe of people to feel safe, comfortable and happy with is a good foundation for mental health.

First and foremost, believe in yourself. Value and love who you are. All the tips, exercises and ideas in this book are to help you do so. You have to feel and see your own value first before others can see it too. When you do, the people with the same values will be attracted to you, making it easier to make genuine friendships. See more on Self Love and Manifesting in on pages 1 and 78.

Think about the things you enjoy that make you feel good about yourself. Then consider what values you want from a friendship, like fun, kindness and respect. Is there something that you could do or join that brings all this together? If so, investigate it further. It is easier to connect with others when they share your interests.

Would it be possible to get a part-time job doing something that interests you? Especially if it is something you were considering as a career when you leave school, though it does not have to be. This provides the opportunity to meet people outside school and become more independent and confident.

For some, sports activities or courses outside of school or work may provide alternative friendships.

Affirmation: *'I am worthy of genuine, fun relationships.'* Say this three times in a row, many times throughout your day for three weeks, or until you feel you no longer need it.

Harry's story

I am 20 years old and have anxiety, which was really bad throughout my teens. To be honest, I didn't really have a social life until Year 12 at high school (age sixteen). I was always a loner because I wasn't sporty but I also wasn't nerdy so I struggled to make friends who were similar to me and understood me. Consequently, I would have a lot of online friends I would talk to, where I felt like I had real relationships. My mum and dad never really understood this, and I agree that it is hard to understand without having online friends yourself, but they were real friendships to me. The people online were there for me when people in real life weren't. Now, I am very fortunate to have both online and real life friends, which I appreciate very much.

One thing that actually helped my social life was seeing a psychologist. They suggested I join social groups or ask friends to hang out and I finally gained the courage to do so (even if reluctantly). I had been so used to being by myself that I didn't entirely know what it was like to have a real friendship. I am so happy now that I did listen to the people telling me to make friends because although I'm not close with all those people I originally invited to hang out with, it allowed me to gain enough confidence to have two very close friends along with others!

World affairs

If you are feeling fearful due to, or for, the state of the world — conflicts, terror attacks, climate change, reducing resources such as fossil fuels and so on — I encourage you to try the following:

Take a short break from looking at news or social media platforms that negatively feed into your mental health. Keep your interests to your local community. After a while, check in with yourself to see how you are feeling. If feeling good and you want to go back to looking at current affairs and events, then do so in small bite-sized ways, checking your feelings as you go.

Look up ways you can help your community. For example, join a project that is cleaning up the local beach, river or park; take part in voluntary work in your neighbourhood, looking after young or elderly people or animals; or look at ways to recycle or reduce buying clothes you will not wear much, and try hiring an outfit rather than buying and discarding it.

Empower your voice. Take part in a peaceful organized rally.

When worrying over the planet, get outside in nature as often as possible. Nature reminds us how magnificent our planet is.

Affirmation: *'I choose to remain calm about our planet. It has been here long before us and works in miraculous ways.'* Say this three times in a row, many times throughout your day for three weeks, or until you feel you no longer need it as you feel calm about the planet.

FINAL THOUGHTS

33.

Ten Quick Daily Hacks

Regardless of what is causing any type of mental health concern, it is usually fear based. It is worth noting, fear is normal — it reminds us to start using our coping strategies and tools.

The following tools are like mindful hacks, designed to settle uneasy feelings. They're not about trying to change everything in your life, but just that moment to help you move forward. You can always take time later to reflect on your feelings when you have the appropriate time, or when feeling up to doing so.

Hack 1

Our thoughts only hurt us if we give them permission to do so by engaging with them. They may not even be true, as sometimes fear is not rational. Try not to label them, over-analyse them or hold onto them — just let them fade. They are just thoughts, nothing more, nothing less.

'Don't chase after thoughts and don't push them away. Let them come in and go out like a swinging door.'

—JAKUSO KWONG

Hack 2

When a worry occurs, set a specific time in three days when you will deal with it. This takes the pressure off in the present moment, allowing you to get on with your day. Most likely, by the time the date arrives, the worry will have been resolved or is no longer important. If it is still relevant, you will then have the appropriate time to deal with it.

Hack 3

Rejection is protection! Think of it as redirecting you to something better.

If you are facing rejection, it is okay to feel upset about it. Feel the feelings, but don't hold onto them — let them recede. Choose to believe you are being redirected somewhere else that will be better suited to you. This way, your focus is on something positive rather than negative.

Hack 4

Day dreaming or fantasizing about happy situations keeps us feeling positive, as happy hormones are released in the body. However, when we fantasize about worrying scenarios, our mind still follows those stressful thoughts and releases stress hormones, regardless of whether the threat is real or not. Stress hormones alter our physical, mental and emotional wellbeing, which is okay when we face imminent danger, but they can be detrimental over a long period of time.

Our brain always looks for evidence to confirm the story in our mind. If that story is saying everything is hard, bad or hopeless, then our brain is going to cherry pick everything in our lives that reinforces that story.

Pause and reflect. Validate whether the threat or scenario is real or whether it is your mind fantasizing. If it is not real or relevant, game over. Shake it off and focus on something else.

Hack 5

Always get as much information as you can on a situation before your brain spins a story based on old knowledge. It is always predicting and formulating your possible future and outcomes based on your past. If information is no longer relevant or it is lacking, this can set up uncertainty.

Hack 6

When worrying, ask yourself one of the following questions:

> 'Is this thought useful? Is it helping me or hurting me?'
>
> 'Does this thought get me closer to where I want to be or is it taking me further away?'
>
> 'Are these thoughts motivating me to move forward or are they blocking me with fear and self-doubt?'
>
> Most likely, the answer will be that it's not helpful and it's stopping you from being happy. Once you are aware of this, this is your cue to do something different. A change of scene helps shift your focus and, thereby, your thoughts. Do something different: go and play with the dog, bake some cookies, shoot some hoops, watch a funny movie — anything that helps shift your thoughts in that moment.

Hack 7

Focus on what you want, rather than what you do not. Your thoughts and feelings follow wherever and whatever your mind is focusing on. Focusing on what you want keeps you moving towards it.

If you focus on something you are trying to avoid, you are elevating it in your mind and your brain will always respond to this. You know what happens when someone says to you, 'Don't trip up' or 'Don't look now.'

By focusing on obstacles, that's all you will see, creating a life filled with them. By focusing on what you want, you will start creating the life you desire.

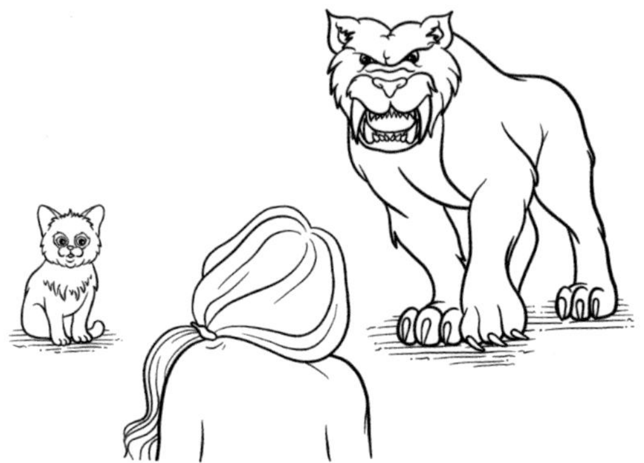

FOCUS ON WHAT YOU WANT IN YOUR LIFE, NOT WHAT YOU DON'T

Hack 8

We constantly critique and judge ourselves. It is best to let go of expectations and judgements, as being hard on yourself doesn't achieve anything and it's a bad idea to be your own worst enemy.

A key way to stop a new experience from causing you to feel disheartened, or from becoming a trigger for future concerns, is to practise surrendering.

This is the balance between working towards what you want, while not being fixated or set in your ways about the outcome and how to achieve it.

Allowing your thoughts and feelings to be *fluid* provides the opportunity for your expectations and life to be the same, and thus, becoming your own best friend.

If not, this can lead to disappointment or frustration, leaving you feeling concerned, annoyed or discouraged. *Move with acceptance and learning rather than expectation and judgement.*

'Let yourself become that space that welcomes any experience without judgement.'

—TSOKNYI RINPOCHE

Hack 9

Life contains all types of experiences. We need those contrasting emotions, situations and experiences to understand their opposite.

When you experience disappointment, sorrow or loss, you can fully appreciate contentment, happiness and success. The joy of riding a bike downhill has to be paid for by first cycling uphill. All energy strives to be in balance and harmony and everything evolves. Know that challenging times will pass, as life continually has its evolving, contrasting ups and downs.

'I'm just gonna say, if there was no Batman, there'd be no Puddin'. Thank you Batman.'

—HARLEY QUINN

Hack 10

If someone has unjustified anger towards you, rather than feeling offended, hurt or upset, ask them if they're okay, as sometimes they are acting this way due to someone or something else that has upset them. If you do this, their anger towards you should dissipate, as they realise it's misplaced.

Create a box that has a lid you can take off easily, called the *Worry Box*. Every time you have a worry, write it on a small piece of paper and pop it into the box. Set a time every day that you will review the contents, like at 5 p.m. every night. Take out each piece of paper and read it. If the worry is still of concern, then it goes back in. If the worry is no longer relevant, throw the piece of paper away. Add any new worries as well.

This exercise helps you focus on the present moment of what is and is not relevant for you. If the worry continues to be present for a while, this means action is required. It is time to take a positive stance towards rectifying the situation.

If creating a Worry Box is not your thing, you could simply create a folder in your notes on your phone called Worry Box, and add, change or delete entries each day.

34.

Taking Back Your Power

'Promise me you'll always remember: You're braver than you believe, and stronger than you seem, and smarter than you think.'

—*POOH'S GRAND ADVENTURE* (DISNEY)

No matter what pain or hurt you carry now, what rejection you may be facing, please know that you are deserving and worthy of a happy life and that there is a bigger picture for you than the one you are seeing and feeling right now.

Everything moves on, everything evolves, all situations change and healing comes one day at a time. New opportunities will present themselves to you and life does get better. Whatever you have been through does not define who you are nor who you will be. You have the ability each day to determine who you want to be and how you want to feel.

Life is a journey, not a destination. It is not a place that one arrives at where all troubles suddenly cease and life is great. It is a constant pathway full of discovery that will continue to evolve as you travel along it, refining your beliefs, opinions and thoughts from all the new experiences. There will be many contrasting discoveries, ones filled with adversity and conflict, as well as peace and joy.

Learning to accept this, embracing it all, ultimately provides you with the best tool to help you on your unique, beautiful path.

Mental health disorders are simply *a signal that action is required*. They are an invitation for action. Something needs to be assessed and remedied to bring emotions and thoughts back into neutrality and balance.

This invitation to act may seem daunting, tiring or even impossible. *It is a process, not an instant fix.* A one-degree change in your thinking and actions has the ability to start the

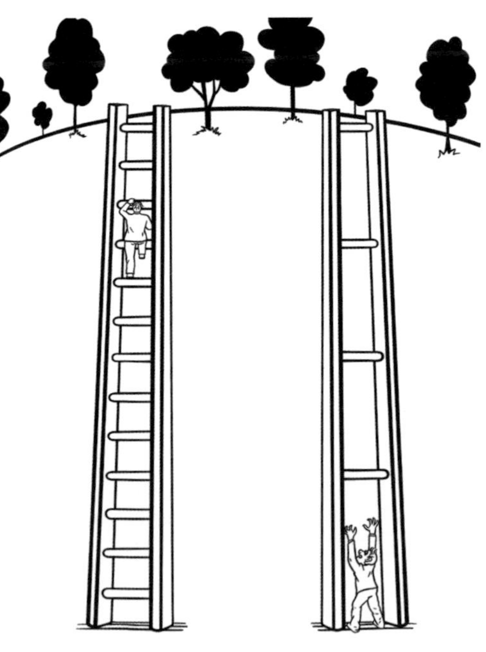

ALL LITTLE STEPS COUNT

process of healing, which ultimately improves anything you choose to focus on.

It's about taking one small positive step at a time, as all baby steps take you towards what you are trying to achieve. Start with something comfortable you can do in a few minutes, regularly throughout each day, creating your little good habits to stabilize your mood. Commit to doing them daily.

Recognize that you are taking back your power, your control of how and who you wish to be that day, as you hold all that power within you. One day at a time. It's worth noting that you do not need to see all those steps and where they may lead — you just need to see and act on that first step and go from there.

Never underestimate the power of small steps! If you were to write one page a day, you could have a novel within a year.

Whether you see a counsellor, psychologist, are on medication to help your mental health or are doing it alone, adding one or more wellbeing habits into your daily routine is your way of taking back control. This is your power, your ability.

All your actions and steps create optimism. Optimism provides a stable emotional foundation for good mental health. As one technique may not work in all situations, be open to trying a few so you may construct your day with the best tools. Using daily little good habits encourages and helps to lock in new positive beliefs and thoughts, and builds resilience against those challenging times.

I will leave you now with my simple philosophy on life which is similar to the Reiki energy healing principles I also teach. In essence, it is living one day at a time, as the past cannot be changed and the future is not yet written, no matter what our thoughts may be telling us!

Wishing you many blessings,

Nic.

Just for today ... BE KIND

Just for today ... BE GRATEFUL

Just for today ... HAVE FUN

Just for today ... TRY NOT TO TAKE MYSELF TOO SERIOUSLY

Just for today ... FOCUS ON WHAT I WANT IN MY LIFE

Acknowledgements

To Sophie and Callum for being my inspiration — you guys rock.

To Steve, my husband, thank you for always supporting and indulging me on my writing path.

Thank you to Lisa Rolle for your encouragement and being my sounding board.

Thanks to Nicola Dodds for saying, 'you should write about young people with anxiety' over that glass of wine — look what happened!!

Thank you to Shannon and Shona for your pearls of wisdom.

Thank you, Georgia Cantlon, for your amazing drawings and helping bring the book to life.

Thank you to the teens who took time to write their stories in the hope to help others — you guys are truly inspirational.

To Kristie, Madeleine and Andrea, my heartfelt gratitude to you all for your professional critiques, insights and recommendations.

A huge thank you to Gareth St John Thomas for helping, advising and encouraging me to keep working on the book, turning it into something that can help teenagers to become their own best friends.

Index

H

I

J

K

L

M

N

O

P

Q

R

S

T

V

W

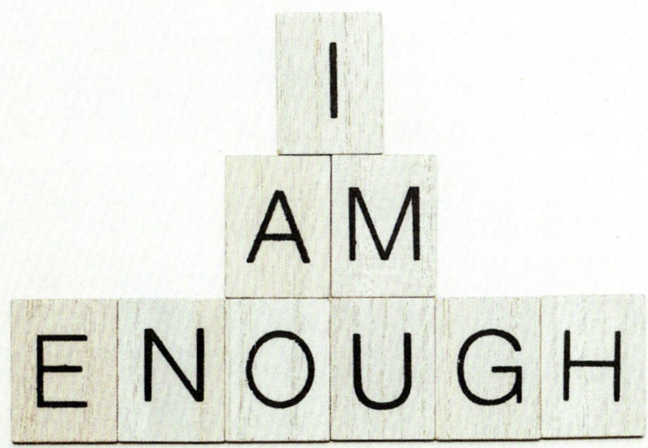
I
AM
ENOUGH